Interdisciplinary Case Management: A Nursing Practice Approach

Shari Garceau

Interdisciplinary Case Management: A Nursing Practice Approach

Springer

Shari Garceau
Austin, TX, USA

ISBN 978-3-032-20959-7 ISBN 978-3-032-20960-3 (eBook)
https://doi.org/10.1007/978-3-032-20960-3

This Springer imprint is published by the registered company Springer Nature Switzerland AG
The registered company address is: Gewerbestrasse 11, 6330 Cham, Switzerland

Preface

Embarking on the journey as a Case Manager has not only been a career choice for me, but it has also been a profoundly fulfilling and transformative experience that has shaped my professional life in countless ways. Each day provides a unique opportunity to make a meaningful difference in the lives of individuals who often find themselves navigating the complexities and challenges of the healthcare system. I am driven not only by my passion for this vital work but also by a deep desire to ignite that same passion in the next generation of case managers. Together, we can propel our profession to new heights, revolutionize the healthcare industry, and emphasize the crucial role each of us plays in enhancing patient outcomes.

Reflecting on my journey, I am continually grateful to my first mentor, whose guidance ignited the spark of my enthusiasm for this field. They provided me with immeasurable wisdom, teaching me the importance of being open to learning and adapting to the unique circumstances and needs of each patient. The ability to recognize when to engage other team members to meet those needs collaboratively is a skill that has proven crucial in my practice. This mentorship not only shaped my professional development but also fostered significant personal growth that continues to inspire me in my work as a Case Manager. It is within this framework of shared knowledge and growth that I firmly believe mentorship plays a pivotal role in our profession. As I advance in my career, I strive to pay it forward by supporting and guiding others who seek to follow a similar path, believing that our collective growth is what will ultimately strengthen the field.

Delving deeper into the nuances of our profession reveals that Case Management, Care Coordination, Social Work, Transitional Care Management, and Utilization Review are not mere titles or isolated roles. Instead, they form interconnected facets of the intricate fabric of the healthcare system. Each role is essential in ensuring that patients receive the comprehensive care they need, underscoring the truth that no professional can thrive in isolation. We are part of a larger community united by a common commitment to improving lives and enriching patient experiences. The strength of this community thrives through our collective efforts and the organizations and certifications that foster an invaluable sense of camaraderie and support among us.

As we look toward the future of our profession, I firmly believe that our ability to share knowledge, insights, and experiences with one another is fundamental to continued evolution and success. The potential inherent in our field is boundless if we wholeheartedly embrace collaboration as a guiding principle. Imagine a world where every Case Manager feels empowered to build upon the knowledge they have gained over time, continuously adapting it to fit the ever-evolving landscape of healthcare. Envision them passing it on to others in ways that create lasting impacts, enabling future professionals to benefit from our shared experiences. This is the vision I cherish and hold close to my heart, one that inspires me to take active steps toward turning it into a reality.

To embark on this transformative journey of empowerment and knowledge sharing, I recognize that the first essential step is to distill the wealth of knowledge I have accumulated throughout my career into written form. By sharing my insights and experiences with the broader community, I hope to illustrate both the challenges and triumphs we face within our field, ultimately illuminating paths for others who are just beginning their careers or seeking to enhance their existing practices. I aim to create resources that serve as guides, bridging gaps in understanding while providing practical tools and insights that can be readily implemented in real-world situations.

As we journey along this shared path, I fervently urge everyone to fully embrace the power of collaboration. Let us take the time to share our stories, lessons learned, and best practices, fostering an environment of openness that encourages growth and development. Together, we can build a robust and unified community of professionals dedicated not only to elevating patient care but also to transforming the healthcare industry on an even larger scale. It is through our collective passion, unwavering commitment, and shared experiences that we can initiate significant and lasting change, one patient at a time.

The impact we can achieve collectively is made even more powerful when we consider the potential ripple effects of our efforts. When we empower and elevate one another, we not only uplift our own experiences but also create a system in which patients benefit from our collaborative work. Every interaction, every decision made in the best interests of our patients has the potential to resonate throughout their lives, affecting families and communities in profound ways. When we strive to enhance the quality of care we deliver and prioritize the patient experience, we are contributing to a healthcare system that not only treats illness but also promotes wellness, prevention, and holistic healing.

I invite all current and future case managers to join me in inspiring one another to rise to the occasion and craft a brighter future for our profession. By committing to work in collaboration, sharing our knowledge, and supporting one another through both challenges and triumphs, we can foster an environment of continuous improvement that ultimately enhances the quality of care we provide. Our journey in this pivotal field extends far beyond individual achievements; it is about uplifting one another and ensuring that every patient in our care receives the utmost support and compassion. Let us embark on this journey together, making a collective impact on the healthcare community that resonates for generations to come. Together, we can be the change that leads us toward a brighter, more innovative future in Case Management.

Case Management is a collaborative process of assessment, planning, facilitation, care coordination, evaluation, and advocacy for options and services to meet an individual's and family's comprehensive health needs through communication and available resources to promote patient safety, quality of care, and cost-effective outcomes.—CMSA Standards of Practice

Utilizing Case Management skills, you can help guarantee that patients receive high-quality and appropriate care and that providers are correctly reimbursed for services that meet the patient's needs. This will lead to optimal clinical and financial outcomes.—Unknown

Austin, NY, USA **Shari Garceau**

Acknowledgments

The evolution of case management has been a dynamic and essential aspect of healthcare delivery, reflecting the growing complexity of patient needs and the intricacies of the healthcare system itself. As healthcare continues to transform, the responsibilities of case managers have expanded significantly, establishing them as pivotal players in bridging gaps, enhancing care coordination, and ensuring that patients receive the appropriate services at the right time.

Case management is fundamentally about integrating healthcare services to meet the unique needs of individuals, particularly those with chronic conditions or complex medical histories. The role involves assessing patients' needs, planning comprehensive care strategies, coordinating resources, and advocating on behalf of patients to navigate the sometimes overwhelming landscape of healthcare options. This practice is particularly vital as the healthcare environment becomes increasingly multifaceted due to factors such as technological advances, policy changes, and the growing prevalence of chronic diseases.

According to MCG Health, understanding the historical context of case management sheds light on the critical need for dedicated professionals who excel at navigating the intricacies of patient care. Case managers advocate for individuals while collaborating with diverse teams of healthcare providers, including doctors, nurses, social workers, and therapists (MCG Health, 2024). The foundational work of Linz et al. (1989) highlights how case management has evolved from its early, rudimentary stages into a more structured and multifaceted discipline. This evolution has led to the establishment of standardized practices that improve patient care and streamline healthcare delivery.

The importance of case management is further emphasized by the resources provided by organizations such as the American Case Management Association (ACMA) and the Case Management Society of America (CMSA). These organizations play a significant role in the ongoing education and certification of case managers, who are integral to maintaining high standards in the field. They offer a wealth of resources, including training programs, professional development opportunities, and forums for networking among practitioners. Access to such knowledge can empower case managers to adopt best practices and incorporate innovative strategies into their work, ultimately improving patient outcomes (American Case Management Association; Case Management Society of America, 2024).

A comprehensive understanding of case management also requires familiarity with the regulatory frameworks that govern it. The Conditions for Coverage (CfCs) and Conditions of Participation (CoPs) established by the Centers for Medicare & Medicaid Services (CMS) delineate the standards necessary for providing adequate care. These regulations ensure that case managers and healthcare facilities adhere to the highest quality of service. Case managers must be well-versed in these regulations, as non-compliance can adversely impact not only the patients they serve but also the healthcare institutions for which they work (CMS, 2024).

Specific resources, such as the "Transitional Care Management Services," highlight the critical role case managers play in facilitating smooth transitions for patients. Transitional care is especially crucial in rural settings, where access to healthcare services may be limited. In such areas, case managers are often tasked with ensuring that patients do not fall through the cracks during transitions between care settings, such as from a hospital to home or from one provider to another (Transitional Care Management Services; Rural Health Information Hub, 2024). Effective transitional care can reduce hospital readmission rates and enhance patient satisfaction, underscoring the value of skilled case management.

As we delve deeper into the intricacies of case management, it becomes imperative to appreciate the historical context, current practices, and ongoing development of this profession. Case management is not just a function of healthcare delivery but is also a response to the evolving demands of society. With rising healthcare costs and the burden of chronic illness on the healthcare system, the need for effective case management will continue to grow.

The advent of technology and the digitization of health records have transformed the landscape of case management. Electronic Health Records (EHRs) or Electronic Medical Records (EMRs) allow case managers to access patient information more efficiently, enabling better coordination of care. The integration of telehealth services also presents new opportunities for case managers to interact with patients remotely, facilitating care for those who may have difficulty accessing services in person. This shift reflects a broader trend toward patient-centered care that prioritizes individual needs and preferences.

The incorporation of data analytics in case management also holds promise for enhancing patient outcomes. By analyzing patient data, case managers can identify trends, predict potential challenges, and tailor interventions more effectively. These insights can lead to more personalized care plans that address specific patient needs, ultimately resulting in improved health outcomes and enhanced patient satisfaction.

As the healthcare landscape continues to evolve, it is crucial for case managers to remain adaptable and continually seek out opportunities for education and professional growth. This mindset will prepare them to address the challenges of an ever-changing environment, including new regulatory requirements, shifts in patient demographics, and evolving patient needs.

In addition to ongoing education and training, case managers must also hone their skills in communication and collaboration. As multifaceted team players within the healthcare system, effective communication is crucial for fostering cooperation among healthcare providers. Case managers must facilitate discussions, share pertinent information, and clarify roles to ensure that each member of the care team understands their contributions to the patient's overall well-being.

This textbook aims to provide a comprehensive overview of the field of case management, drawing on the insights of contemporary experts and detailed studies that inform the evolving practice. By examining the historical development, current frameworks, and future challenges, this resource seeks to prepare professionals for the complexities that lie ahead in case management. Understanding the past and present dynamics of case management will equip practitioners with the knowledge needed to navigate an increasingly intricate healthcare landscape, ultimately enhancing the quality of care delivered to patients across diverse settings.

Integrating the perspectives presented in this textbook will not only foster a deeper appreciation for the vital role of case management but also encourage practitioners to remain committed to excellence in their practice. As the profession continues to evolve, ongoing discussions about best practices, innovative strategies, and collaboration among stakeholders will be essential in addressing the persistent challenges faced by healthcare systems today. Together, we can ensure that case management will continue to adapt and thrive, ultimately leading to better health outcomes and improved quality of life for patients and their families.

Embarking on this transformative journey of empowerment and knowledge sharing fills me with a deep sense of purpose and gratitude for those who shared their passion for the role of Case Management with me. I recognize that the first crucial step in this process is to carefully distill the wealth of experiences and insights I have gained throughout my career into written form. By sharing these reflections with the broader community, I hope to shed light on both the challenges and triumphs we encounter in our field.

My goal is to create resources that resonate with those who are just beginning their careers and those who are striving to enhance their existing practices. I believe that by bridging gaps in understanding, I can provide practical tools and insights that can be readily applied in real-world situations. Together, we can foster a spirit of collaboration, growth, and mutual support, empowering each other to navigate our paths with confidence and purpose. Ultimately, my aim is to contribute to a vibrant and interconnected community that inspires and uplifts every current and future Case Manager.

Contents

1 Overview of Case Management 1
1.1 History of Case Management 3
1.2 Integration into Healthcare Settings 4
1.3 Case Management Models in Healthcare 8
1.4 Collaborative Roles of Nurses and Social Workers 9
1.5 The Dyad Model: Balancing Utilization Review and Discharge Planning 9
1.6 The Triad Model: Enhancing Collaboration and Care Quality 10
1.7 Role of Non-Licensed Staff 11

2 Regulations and Compliance Impacting Case Management 13
2.1 Conditions of Participation 14
Utilization Review 14
Discharge Planning and Conflict of Interest 14
Social Drivers of Health (SDoH) and Health-Related Social Needs (HRSN) 16
Patient Rights (as Applies to Case Management Roles) 16
Choice of Providers (Freedom of Choice) 18
Informed Decisions About Care 18
Advance Directives 19
Family Notification 19
Privacy and Safety 19
Access to Records 19
Freedom from Abuse 20
Right to Appeal 20
Utilization Management Committee (UMC) 20
2.2 CMS Forms and Requirements 21
Two Midnight Rule (2MN) 21
Condition Code 44 (Including Medicare Outpatient Observation Notice and Medicare Change in Status Notification) 21
Important Message from Medicare (IMM) 23
Recertification and Extended Stay Review 23
Hospital Issued Notice of Noncoverage (HINN) 24

2.3 Patient Protection and Complaint Investigation 25
Office of the Inspector General (OIG) 25
Beneficiary and Family Centered Care – Quality Improvement Organization (BFCC-QIO) 25
2.4 Facility Accreditation 26
Auditing/Survey Agencies 26
2.5 Case Studies 27
Two-Midnight Rule 27
References 28

3 Case Management Settings 29
3.1 The Foundation of Case Management 30
3.2 The Role of Technology 30
3.3 Coordination Across Healthcare Settings 31
3.4 Collaboration with Payors 31
3.5 Care Navigation and the Role of the Navigation Nurse or Social Worker 32
3.6 Special Populations and Specific Needs 32
3.7 Education and Training for Future Generations 33
3.8 The Evolving Future of Case Management 33
3.9 Adapting to Change 34
3.10 Case Study 34
Coordination Across the Healthcare Continuum 34
Does this communication potentially impact patient care? 35

4 Roles of the Utilization Review Team 37
4.1 Point of Entry Utilization Management 39
Point of Entry: Surgical and Procedural Areas 40
Point of Entry: Transfer 42
Point of Entry: Direct Admission 42
Point of Entry: Admission via the Emergency Department or Free-standing Emergency Centers 43
4.2 Important Role for Utilization Review Integration 44
4.3 Financial Impact on Patients and Facilities 45
4.4 Observation Management 45
4.5 Expanding on Focused Observation Rounds 47
4.6 Implementing Rapid Observation Rounds 48
4.7 Strengthening Inpatient Utilization Management 48
4.8 Coordinating with Other Teams 49
4.9 The Role of Collaboration in Clinical Documentation Integrity (CDI) 49
4.10 Strategic Coordination with the Care Team 50
4.11 Enhancing Team Collaboration 50
4.12 Continuous Improvement and Adaptation 51
4.13 Denial Management 51
4.14 Short Stay Review 52

4.15 Utilization Review is a Key Member of the Revenue Cycle Team...... 53
4.16 Payor Relations.. 55
4.17 Case Studies.. 55
Observation Management.. 55
Patient Without Medical Necessity Criteria.. 56
Denial Appeal.. 56

5 Roles Within Case Management to Support Patient Throughput 59
5.1 Nurse Case Manager Role.. 60
5.2 Social Worker Role.. 61
5.3 Collaboration Between Roles.. 61
5.4 Supporting Patients Across the Continuum of Care.. 62
5.5 Discharge Planning.. 63
5.6 Care Coordination.. 64
5.7 Readmission Risk Management.. 65
5.8 Readmission Risk Mitigation.. 66
5.9 Readmission Assessment After Readmission.. 67
5.10 Patient Throughput Management and Bed Capacity Management.... 68
Length of Stay Management.. 68
Length of Stay Outlier Management.. 69
High-Risk for Length of Stay Outlier Identification.. 70
Length of Stay Outlier High-Level Management.. 71
Long Stay Management of Custodial Cases.. 72
5.11 Avoidable Days and Delays.. 73
5.12 Avoidable Days and Delays Cause-Specific.. 74
Patient/Family Barriers.. 74
Clinical Complex Care Cases.. 75
External Provider Barriers.. 76
Internal/System Barriers.. 76
Payor Barriers.. 77
Provider Barriers.. 78
5.13 Patient Care Rounds.. 78
5.14 Daily Rounds on Medical/Surgical Units.. 79
5.15 Daily Rounds for Intensive Care Units.. 80
5.16 Discharge Care Team Huddles.. 81
5.17 Transitional Care (TC) and Population Health.. 83
5.18 Targeted Case Management (TCM).. 84
5.19 Community Liaison.. 86
5.20 Case Manager as Educator.. 87
5.21 Case Studies.. 88
Readmission Prevention.. 88
Multidisciplinary Rounds and Complex Case.. 89

6 Reporting and Monitoring.. 91
6.1 Compliance.. 91
6.2 Key Performance Indicators.. 93

6.3 Physician Advisor Engagement ... 94
6.4 Case Management Value Reflected in Data ... 94

7 Case Management as a Profession ... 97

8 Looking to the Future ... 101
8.1 Artificial Intelligence (AI) and Automation in Case Management ... 102

9 Workflows ... 105
9.1 UM, CM, CDI Communication ... 107
9.2 Utilization Management Process Workflows ... 108
High-Level Utilization Management Function ... 108
Initial Review ... 109
Initial Review from the Logistic (Transfer) Center or Direct Admit ... 110
Pre-Procedural ... 111
Pre-Procedure Review and Discharge Assessment ... 112
Post-Procedure ... 113
Observation/Outpatient in a Bed Management ... 114
MOON Process ... 115
Condition Code 44 ... 116
Concurrent Review ... 117
Short-Stay Review ... 118
Occurrence Span Code 72 ... 119
Commercial Downgrade ... 120
Denial Management ... 121
Hospital-Issued Notice of Noncoverage (HINN 1) ... 122
Hospital-Issued Notice of Noncoverage (HINN 10) ... 123
Hospital-Issued Notice of Noncoverage (HINN 11) ... 124
Notice of Noncoverage (Not Acute Care Hospital Setting) ... 125
QIO Request for Records ... 125
9.3 Case Management Process Workflows ... 127
Important Message from Medicare (IMM) ... 127
Discharge Appeal ... 128
9.4 Hospital-Issued Notice of Noncoverage (HINN 12) ... 129
High-Level CM Daily Process ... 130
Unfunded Patient Screening ... 131
Readmission Risk/Readmission Mitigation ... 132
Readmission Follow-Up ... 133
Discharge Assessment ... 134
Discharge Simple vs Complex ... 135
Long-Stay High Risk Identification ... 136
MDR/PPR/IDT ... 137
Long-Stay Rounds ... 138
Length of Stay Outlier—Non-Custodial ... 139

Length of Stay Outlier—Custodial . . . 140
Declining Discharge Escalation . . . 141
Post-Acute Provider Discharge. . . . 142
Transitional Care . . . 143
Avoidable Delay/Day High-Level . . . 144
Avoidable Delay—Patient or Family Barrier. . . . 145
Avoidable Delay Potential—Complex Care . . . 146
Avoidable Delay/Day—External. . . . 147
Avoidable Delay/Day—Internal . . . 148
Avoidable Delay/Day—Provider. . . . 149
Avoidable Delay/Day—Payor . . . 150

10 Educational Tip Sheets . . . 151
10.1 Conditions of Participation (CoP) Tip Sheet . . . 152
What Are the Conditions of Participation? . . . 152
What Conditions of Participation Apply to Utilization Management? . . . 153
What Is the Value of the Conditions of Participation? . . . 153
10.2 Conflict of Interest Tip Sheet . . . 153
What Is Considered Conflict of Interest? . . . 153
What Is the Stark Law? . . . 154
What Is the Value of the Reviewing Conflict of Interest? . . . 154
10.3 Utilization Management Committee Tip Sheet . . . 154
Who Are the Participants of the UR Committee?. . . . 154
How Often and Where Does the UR Committee Meet?. . . . 155
What Does the UR Committee Discuss? . . . 155
What Is the Value of the Utilization Review Committee?. . . . 155
10.4 Two-Midnight Rule Tip Sheet . . . 155
How Was the Two-Midnight Rule Developed?. . . . 155
What Is the Basic Principle of the Two-Midnight Rule?. . . . 156
Are There Exclusions from the Two-Midnight Rule? . . . 156
How Are Audits Viewed By CMS? . . . 156
What Is the Value of the Two-Midnight Rule? . . . 156
10.5 Condition Code 44 (CC44) Tip Sheet. . . . 156
What Are Documentation Requirements for a CC 44? . . . 157
What Must Be Considered Prior to a CC 44? . . . 157
What Are the Steps for the Physician and Facility in the CC 44 Process? . . . 157
What Is the Value in a Condition Code 44? . . . 157
10.6 Occurrence Span Code 72 Tip Sheet . . . 158
How Does Utilization Management Identify Accounts to Be Billed with Occurrence Code 72? . . . 158

What Services Count Towards an Occurrence Span Code 72? 158
What Is the Value of the Occurrence Span Code 72? 158
10.7 Important Message from Medicare (IMM) Tip Sheet 158
What Received the Important Message from Medicare Notices? 159
What Is the Important Message from Medicare and Detailed Notice of Discharge? 159
When Do These Notices Need to Be Given? 159
What Role Does Case Management/Utilization Management Play in the Process? 159
What Is the Value of the Important Message? 160
10.8 Medicare Outpatient Observation Notice (MOON) Tip Sheet 160
What Is Considered Outpatient Observation Services? 160
Are There Guidelines for the Notification? 160
What Is Covered in Under the Medicare Outpatient Observation Notice? 161
What Is the Value of MOON? 161
10.9 Hospital-Issued Notice of Noncoverage (HINN) Tip Sheet 161
Are There Times When a HINN Is Not Appropriate? 162
What Is the Purpose of a HINN? 162
What Are the Conditions Included in the HINN Process? 162
What Is the Value of the HINN Process? 162
10.10 CMS Inpatient Only List (Addendum E) Tip Sheet 162
What Is the Difference with Other Resource Inpatient Only Lists? 163
What Should Utilization Management Do When Reviewing Surgical Cases? 163
Why Is the Inpatient Only List important? 163
10.11 Transforming Episode Accountability Modes (TEAM) Tip Sheet 163
Is Participation in the TEAMS Model Mandatory? 163
What Patients Will Be Included as Part of the TEAM Model? 164
What Services Are Included in the 90-Day TEAM Model? 164
What Is the Physician Role in the TEAM Model? 164
What Is the Value of the TEAM Model? 164
10.12 Bundled Payments for Care Improvement (BPCI) Tip Sheet 165
What Patients Will Be Part of BPCI? 165
What Services are Included in the 90-Day BPCI Program? 165
What Is the Physician Role in BCPI? 166
What Is Case Managements Role in BPCI? 166
Essential to the Success of the BPCI Program Is a Safe, Timely Discharge Plan 166
Is There Anything New Required as Part of BPCI? 166
What Is the Value of the Bundled Payment for Care Improvement Program? 167

10.13 Utilization Review Tip Sheet 167
How Do We Use Information from a Utilization Review? 167
What Is the Review Process?. 167
What Is the Value of the Utilization Review Process?. 168
10.14 Procedural Utilization Management Tip Sheet. 168
What Is Procedural Utilization Management? 168
What Can We Do to Manage Procedural Cases Optimally?. 168
What Is the Value of Procedural Utilization Management? 169
10.15 Concurrent Review Tip Sheet. 169
What Is Concurrent Review Utilization Management? 169
What Can We Do to Manage Concurrent Cases?. 169
What Is the Value of Concurrent Review Utilization Management? 170
10.16 Extended Stay Review Tip Sheet 170
How Do We Manage Extended Stay Cases? 170
Why Do We Want to Manage Length of Stay? 170
10.17 Emergency Department Utilization Management Tip Sheet 171
What Can We Do to Improve ED Admissions? 171
What Can Utilization Management to for the Facility as Part of the Emergency Department?. 171
What Is the Value of Utilization Management in the Emergency Department?. 171
10.18 Transfer Center and Direct Admit Tip Sheet 171
What Is Role of Review Utilization Management? 172
What Can Utilization Management Do to Support Transfer Center and Direct Admit Cases? 172
What Is the Value of Utilization Management in Logistics Center and Direct Admits?. 172
10.19 Observation Management Tip Sheet. 172
What Is Observation?. 173
What Can We Do to Manage Observation Cases? 173
What Is the Value of Observation Management?. 173
10.20 Outpatient in a Bed Management Tip Sheet. 173
What Is Outpatient in a Bed? 174
What Can We Do to Manage Outpatient in a Bed cases?. 174
What Is the Value of Outpatient in a Bed Management? 174
10.21 Physician Advisor (PA) Tip Sheet 175
What Is the Physician Advisor Role? 175
What Does a Physician Advisor Do? 175
What Is the Value of a Physician Advisor Program?. 175
10.22 Denial Management Tip Sheet 176
How Can Utilization Management Prevent a Denial? 176

What Is a Concurrent Denial and What Can Utilization Management Do to Mitigate? 176
What Will Following a Denial Management Process Accomplish? 176
10.23 Short-Stay Inpatient Management Tip Sheet 176
Is the Inpatient Level of Care Billing Valid? 177
What Is the CMS Policy Regarding Length of Stays Expected to be Less than Two Midnights? 177
What Is the Value of Reviewing Short-Stay Inpatient Accounts? 177
10.24 Interrater Reliability Tip Sheet 177
What Is Reviewed Using Interrater Reliability? 178
Why Is the Interrater Reliability Audit Performed? 178
What Is the Value of Interrater Reliability Audits? 178
10.25 Care Coordination Tip Sheet 178
What Is Care Coordination? 178
How Can We Coordinate Care for Our Patients? 179
Who Is Part of Care Coordination? 179
What Is the Value of Care Coordination? 179
10.26 Multidisciplinary Rounds (MDR)/Patient Progression Rounds (PPR)/Interdisciplinary Team (IDT) Tip Sheet 179
What Is the Purpose of the MDR? 180
Who Are the Participants in the Multidisciplinary Team? 180
What Does the Multidisciplinary Team discuss? 180
What Is the Value of the Interdisciplinary Team? 180
10.27 Resource Management Tip Sheet 180
What Is Resource Management? 180
What Areas Are included in Resource Management? 181
What Is the Value of Resource Management? 181
10.28 Discharge Planning Tip Sheet 181
What Is the Value of Discharge Planning? 182
10.29 Discharge Planning: Home Health (HH) Tip Sheet 182
What Can Be Managed by Home Health Care? 182
What Should Be Expected from Home Health Care? 182
What Is the Benefit of Home Health? 183
10.30 Discharge Planning: Hospice Tip Sheet 183
What Qualifies for Hospice Care? 183
What Services Are Offered by Hospice? 183
Where Can Hospice Services Be Provided? 184
What Are the Benefits of Understanding Hospice? 184
10.31 Discharge Planning: Acute Inpatient Rehabilitation (IRF/ARF) Tip Sheet 185
What Patients Benefit from Acute Inpatient Rehab Level of Care? 186
What Are the Requirements for Acute Rehabilitation Services? 186
What Diagnoses Meet CMS Criteria? 186

What Are the Benefits of Understanding Acute Rehab? 186
10.32 Discharge Planning: Long Term Acute Care (LTAC) Tip Sheet. . . . 187
What Is Managed by Long-Term Acute Care Level of Care? 187
What Are the Requirements for Long-Term Acute Care Services? 187
What Are the Benefits of Understanding LTAC? 187
10.33 Length of Stay Alphabet Tip Sheet. 188
What Is Length of Stay Optimization? 188
What Are the Acronyms and What Do They Mean? 188
10.34 Length of Stay Tip Sheet 189
Why Does the Hospital Want to Optimize Each Patient's Length of Stay? 189
How Can We Optimize Length of Stay? 189
Who Is Needed for a Partnership to Assist with Throughput? 189
10.35 Length of Stay Optimization Tip Sheet 190
How Can We Optimize Length of Stay for Each Patient? 190
What Is a Process for Reviewing Extended (Outlier) Cases? 191
What Is the Benefit of Length of Stay Management? 191
10.37 Avoidable Delay/Day Tip Sheet 191
Why Do We Document Avoidable Days/Delays? 191
Where Is Information Regarding Avoidable/Denied Days Documented? 191
What Documentation Should Be Included? 192
Who Receives Documentation? 192
10.37 Readmission Management Tip Sheet 192
What Is a Hospital Readmission? 192
What Are the Impacts of Hospital Readmissions? 193
How Can Readmission Rates Be Lowered?. 193
What Is the Value of Reducing Readmissions? 193
10.38 Supporting Patients with Behavioral Health Issues Tip Sheet 193
What Causes Increased Stress and Decreased Coping in Patients with Behavioral Health History? 194
How Can We Reduce Stress for This Population? 194

11 Conclusion 195

About the Author

Shari Garceau is an experienced registered nurse (RN) with over 20 years of experience in the healthcare field, specializing in case management, utilization review, revenue cycle, clinical documentation, quality, risk, and process improvements for more than 15 years. She is a strategic leader who has successfully restructured case management and utilization review departments across various healthcare systems.

Her active involvement with the American Case Management Association (ACMA) and the Case Management Society of America (CMSA) underscores her dedication to improving patient care and advocating for coverage benefits through healthcare legislation. Shari is known for her compassionate and collaborative approach, excelling in clinical documentation analysis, staff education, and fostering teamwork among case management personnel.

As a subject matter expert in case management, care coordination, utilization review, revenue cycle management, payor relations, quality, and risk, she has a proven ability to identify and implement process improvements that align with quality and compliance standards. Shari has also taken on roles as a Centers for Medicare & Medicaid Services (CMS) compliance officer and lead educator, developing onboarding and continuing education programs to prepare healthcare facilities for regulatory surveys.

Her comprehensive experience and dedication enable her to effectively lead teams and elevate the standards of care within the healthcare industry.

Overview of Case Management

1

Learning Objectives

1. **Understand the foundational concepts:** Gain a clear understanding of the basic principles and key terms related to Case Management.
2. **Identify the scope and significance:** Recognize the importance and relevance of the role within the healthcare system.
3. **Explore historical background:** Learn about the history and evolution of Case Management and its many roles.
4. **Develop critical thinking skills:** Apply critical thinking to the concepts surrounding the role.
5. **Apply introductory knowledge:** Begin to apply the concepts learned to real-world scenarios and examples.

This textbook serves as a guide, offering a comprehensive foundation for establishing and implementing best practices within the realm of Case Management. Whether the terminology used for the role of coordinating care for patients across the continuum of care has alternated between Case Management and Care Management over the years, but the role remains consistent. The workflow processes outlined herein form a fundamental framework that can be tailored to address the unique needs of your specific facility or organization. While this text covers many widely accepted and practiced methodologies under the Case Management umbrella, it is important to note that it is not exhaustive. The field of Case Management is dynamic, characterized by a continual evolution influenced by emerging responsibilities, changing regulations, and a growing awareness of patient-centered care. This ongoing evolution is one of the most exciting aspects of Case Management, encompassing diverse roles across the healthcare landscape.

S. Garceau, *Interdisciplinary Case Management: A Nursing Practice Approach*,
https://doi.org/10.1007/978-3-032-20960-3_1

By leveraging these established workflows, professionals can harness the potential of current and forthcoming technologies to align their practices with both regulatory requirements and industry best practices. Advanced technology can enhance the efficiency of Case Management operations by automating the identification of cases that require attention, managing ongoing cases in accordance with established standards, facilitating referrals to specialized Care Coordination teams, and swiftly pinpointing documentation that might be at risk of denial. These capabilities represent just a few of the numerous ways technology can streamline Case Management processes, allowing professionals to prioritize their caseloads effectively and refine their workflow.

Numerous software programs and systems are already implemented by many Case Managers and Utilization Review teams in various healthcare environments, with an increasing number of solutions still in development. Many of these systems incorporate artificial intelligence (AI) or automation tools, which can review documentation in real time. They provide recommendations for the appropriate level of care and support for critical transition or discharge planning. As we continue to build and refine these systems, we unlock new pathways for enhancing both efficiency and the role of case management, ultimately leading to improved patient care outcomes. However, it is essential to understand that technology should augment, rather than replace, the vital human elements of care.

While embracing technological advancements is essential in this growing field, it is equally critical to maintain a firm commitment to appropriately managing cases and keeping the patient at the heart of all efforts. Patients are our primary focus and the driving force behind our work. As healthcare professionals, Case Managers rely on meaningful personal interactions to accurately gauge patient needs. This engagement enables them to support patients in accessing the right resources and services to address their individual goals for optimal health and well-being effectively. It is through these interactions that Case Managers can better understand the complexities of each patient's circumstances, tailoring interventions and support strategies that resonate with each individual's unique situation.

Case Management is a vital discipline within the healthcare industry, playing a crucial role in ensuring that patients receive the highest quality of care. By coordinating treatment plans and securing the necessary resources and services, case management helps facilitate a seamless journey through the healthcare system. Furthermore, it ensures that healthcare facilities operate efficiently and effectively, all while adhering to regulatory and quality standards. Case Management professionals work hand in hand with patients, healthcare providers, and a range of other stakeholders, ensuring that every patient receives the most appropriate and effective care throughout their healthcare journey. This collaborative approach not only fosters better communication among care team members but also enhances the overall experience for the patient and their family.

The importance of Case Management extends far beyond administrative efficiency—it has significant, far-reaching implications for the healthcare industry as a whole. Effective Case Management not only elevates the standard of care for patients but also fosters a collaborative healthcare environment where all participants work cohesively toward shared goals. By recognizing and responding to the diverse needs of patients, Case Managers position themselves as essential advocates in the healthcare system, influencing both individual outcomes and broader healthcare quality. The ripple effect of informed and empathetic Case Management can reverberate throughout communities, ultimately leading to healthier populations and a more effective healthcare delivery system overall. By committedly pursuing excellence in practice, Case Managers can shape a better future for the healthcare industry and the many individuals it serves.

1.1 History of Case Management

The concept of Case Management has its roots in the early nineteenth century. Still, it was not until the mid-twentieth century that significant regulatory changes in the United States propelled this function into a central role within patient care. Key legislative measures such as the Social Security Act of 1935, the Developmental Disabilities Act of 1974, and the Older Americans Act of 1978 set critical standards and established the framework for a more structured approach to patient management. These acts underscored the necessity for coordinated care, particularly for vulnerable populations, thereby catalyzing the evolution of Case Management as we understand it today.

In its early stages, Case Management primarily concentrated on managing chronic illnesses and controlling healthcare costs. The urgency to streamline medical services arose from the increasing prevalence of chronic conditions and the need for more efficient allocation of healthcare resources. The complexity of managing patients with chronic illnesses highlighted the need for a coordinated approach that brings together various healthcare services and providers. This shift became increasingly important as the understanding of chronic diseases expanded, revealing the multi-faceted support and interventions required to manage these conditions effectively.

Over time, however, the role of Case Management has expanded significantly, transforming into a multi-dimensional profession that is essential for achieving not only positive patient outcomes but also enhancing overall quality of life while meeting the intricate business demands of the healthcare industry. Today's Case Management professionals are tasked with navigating complex healthcare landscapes, ensuring that patients not only receive appropriate medical treatments but also are supported in their overall well-being. This includes addressing social determinants of health, such as housing, education, and access to nutritious food, thereby incorporating a holistic view of patient care.

The collaboration between Case Management (CM) and Clinical Documentation Integrity (CDI) is vital in bridging the gap between clinical teams and administrative functions. This partnership ensures that the best healthcare practices are delivered to patients while simultaneously adhering to business standards that support the financial viability of healthcare providers. Effective communication and collaboration are essential, as Case Managers must be adept at working with various stakeholders, including physicians, nurses, social workers, and insurance representatives, to coordinate care and optimize patient outcomes.

By striking this balance, Case Management practitioners play an integral role in the healthcare ecosystem, underpinning both patient care and organizational performance. They often serve as the linchpin in facilitating communication among all parties involved in a patient's care journey. This role requires a unique skill set, including proficiency in clinical knowledge, empathy, problem-solving capabilities, and negotiation skills. Case Managers must be equipped to handle diverse scenarios that can vary widely in complexity, which often requires ongoing education and training to stay current with best practices and regulatory requirements.

Originally, Case Management was predominantly associated with discharge planning, aiming to guarantee that patients were equipped with the necessary services and supports prior to leaving the healthcare facility. However, this narrow focus has shifted dramatically; today's Case Management encompasses a broad array of responsibilities and skills, reflecting the complexities of contemporary healthcare delivery. The modern Case Manager is involved in ensuring continuity of care from hospital to home, coordinating follow-up appointments, and connecting patients with community resources that can support their ongoing health needs.

Additionally, the advent of technology has greatly influenced the field of Case Management, enabling better tracking and analysis of patient data. Electronic health records (EHR) allow Case Managers to access a patient's history, treatment plans, and progress more efficiently, leading to better-informed decisions. Telehealth and digital communication tools facilitate ongoing interactions with patients, enhancing engagement and adherence to care plans. This technological integration not only streamlines workflows but also empowers patients, giving them greater access to their health information and fostering a partnership in their care.

As the healthcare landscape continues to evolve with value-based care and population health management gaining prominence, the role of Case Management is becoming even more crucial. Practitioners are increasingly involved in assessing risk, identifying barriers to care, and implementing strategies to improve health outcomes on a larger scale. They often engage in quality improvement initiatives that target specific patient populations, aiming to reduce readmission rates and improve chronic disease management.

The history of Case Management is characterized by its transformation from a simple discharge planning function to a vital component of the healthcare delivery system. As it continues to evolve, it remains essential in addressing the complexities of healthcare today, focusing on comprehensive care coordination that meets the diverse needs of patients. Through collaboration with various sectors and the integration of technology, Case Management is poised to play an increasingly important role in the future of healthcare, underlining its impact on patient outcomes and system efficiency. The journey of Case Management reflects a broader commitment within the healthcare system to ensure that all patients receive the holistic, coordinated care they deserve.

1.2 Integration into Healthcare Settings

The significance of Case Management in the healthcare landscape cannot be overstated, particularly as the field continues to evolve rapidly in response to shifting patient needs and technological advancements. A fundamental principle of effective Case Management is maintaining the patient at the heart of care, all while navigating the increasingly intricate business aspects of healthcare delivery. This dual focus not only enhances patient satisfaction but also promotes improved health outcomes.

As we delve deeper into the intricacies of Case Management, it's essential to highlight the vital elements that contribute to its efficacy in healthcare settings. One of the most prominent elements is the acknowledgment of every patient's unique circumstances. Various factors, including socioeconomic status, cultural background, and individual healthcare needs, influence the journey each patient undertakes. Thus, Case Management professionals must adopt a holistic approach, considering these diverse facets when crafting and implementing care plans.

Healthcare leaders are increasingly involving Case Management professionals in strategic decision-making processes. By integrating Case Management leadership into broader organizational discussions, healthcare systems are better equipped to implement initiatives that foster patient-centered care and enhance clinical outcomes. This participatory approach not only empowers Case Managers but also encourages a culture of collaboration among all members of the healthcare team.

The definition of Case Management has adapted to reflect these changes within the healthcare environment. No longer viewed merely as a standalone department or function, Case Management is now regarded as a collaborative team process that operates across the entire continuum of care in various healthcare settings. This paradigm shift emphasizes the importance of teamwork and communication among diverse healthcare professionals, aligning efforts to ensure that patients receive comprehensive, coordinated, and timely care.

In modern healthcare, the role of technology cannot be ignored. Advanced electronic health records (EHRs) and other health information technology solutions have revolutionized the way Case Managers interact with patient data and with one another. These tools enable Case Managers to track patient progress more effectively, share information quickly, and communicate seamlessly with other departments. The integration of these technologies aids in reducing redundancies and preventing errors, ultimately enhancing the overall efficiency of patient care.

The evolving landscape has led to increased emphasis on data analytics in Case Management. Utilizing data to identify trends, monitor outcomes, and evaluate the effectiveness of various interventions allows healthcare organizations to improve their services proactively. By analyzing data patterns, healthcare providers can anticipate challenges and tailor interventions to meet the specific needs of their patient population. This proactive approach not only supports better health outcomes but also helps identify areas for improvement within the healthcare system itself.

As we observe the movement towards value-based care, the role of Case Management grows even more critical. Value-based care emphasizes the quality rather than the quantity of care delivered to patients. Case Managers are key players in this shift, ensuring that patients receive appropriate care tailored to their needs while also focusing on cost-effectiveness. This involves regularly evaluating treatment plans, addressing patient barriers to adherence, and coordinating care across multiple providers to ensure that patients do not fall through the cracks of the healthcare system.

Patient progression is often viewed as a linear process in the hospital setting, typically characterized by three stages (Fig. 1.1):

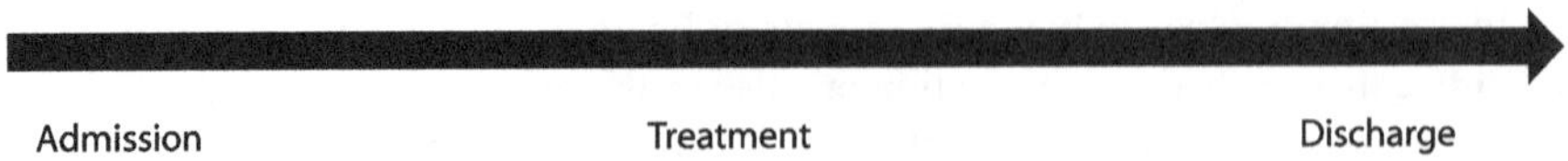

Fig. 1.1 Linear progression of patient progression starting at admission through discharge. Created by the author

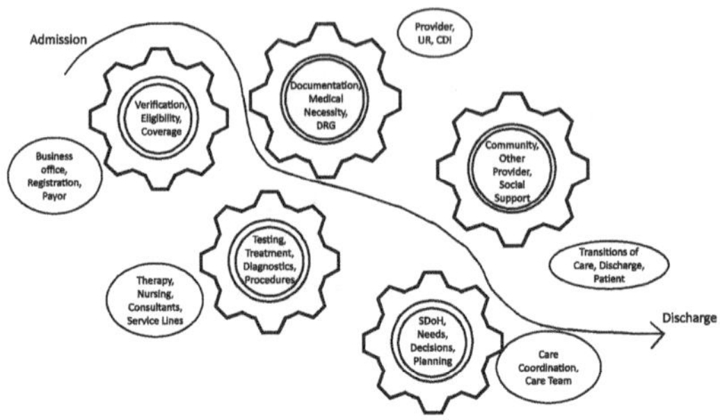

Fig. 1.2 A progression of patient care with the transitions between different members and departments involved in the patient care and treatment. Created by the author

However, this simplistic view fails to capture the complexities involved in patient care. The truth is that patient progression is a multifaceted system designed to ensure that individuals receive optimal care throughout their healthcare journey, from admission to discharge. This journey involves a series of interconnected components, each playing a vital role in shaping the patient experience (Fig. 1.2).

Effective communication among all departments—such as nursing, pharmacy, diagnostics, and case management—is crucial for seamless transitions and timely interventions. It's essential to create an environment where interdisciplinary collaboration is not only encouraged but becomes the norm. Regular multidisciplinary rounds can foster open dialogue between teams, enabling them to address any concerns that may arise in real-time and facilitating a more cohesive care experience for the patient.

When these elements operate in harmony, they facilitate a comprehensive approach to patient care that enhances outcomes and ensures safety. However, if even one component becomes inefficient, it can create bottlenecks that disrupt the flow of services, ultimately delaying patient care and potentially impacting recovery. For instance, delays in obtaining lab results can impede timely diagnosis and treatment, leading to an increased length of stay and potential complications.

In preparation for our upcoming discussion on Case Management, we will explore the intricacies of patient progression in greater detail. We will examine the specific roles and responsibilities of healthcare professionals involved in this process, as well as strategies for optimizing communication and collaboration across departments. By understanding these dynamics, we can better appreciate how to streamline patient care and improve overall healthcare delivery.

Training and education also play a crucial role in ensuring that all healthcare professionals involved in Case Management are equipped to navigate these complexities. Continuous professional development opportunities, including workshops and seminars, can enhance the skills of Case Managers and others in the field. Additionally, mentoring programs can foster knowledge sharing and support new Case Managers as they learn to navigate the healthcare landscape.

As healthcare continues to embrace practices that prioritize patient care, the role of Case Management will undoubtedly remain central to shaping effective patient care strategies and fostering a sustainable healthcare system. The ongoing professional development and integration of Case Management into the broader healthcare delivery framework underscore its pivotal position in transforming patient experiences and achieving better outcomes.

Case Management operates within the confines of healthcare providers as well has within the payor sector of healthcare. The roles of Utilization Management and Case Management provide review of record, coordination of patient benefits, care coordination services for patient populations with chronic illnesses or special healthcare considerations, and coordination with healthcare providers via open and transparent communication.

These two domains work in tandem to ensure the patients receive appropriate, high-quality care while simultaneously managing costs and resource utilization effectively. Within this structure, the roles of Utilization Management and Case Management are distinct yet complementary. Utilization Management primarily involves the systematic review of patient records and medical necessity determinations to ensure that care provided aligns with established best practices and insurance requirements. This review process helps to prevent unnecessary treatments and supports the judicious use of healthcare resources, promoting both cost-effectiveness and patient safety.

Case Management, by contrast, is deeply rooted in care coordination and advocacy, particularly for patient populations with chronic illnesses, special healthcare considerations, or complex social needs. Case Managers serve as liaisons between patients, families, healthcare providers, and insurance entities, ensuring that every aspect of a patient's care plan is communicated clearly and executed efficiently. Their responsibilities include coordinating patient benefits, facilitating access to appropriate care settings, and arranging for specialized services such as home health, rehabilitation, and community resources.

A critical component of Case Management is the proactive identification of at-risk patients who may require more intensive support to achieve optimal health outcomes. Employing data analytics and evidence-based protocols, Case Managers can anticipate potential complications, intervene early to address barriers, and develop individualized care strategies. This population health approach enables organizations to focus on preventive interventions, reducing the likelihood of hospital readmissions, emergency department visits, and unnecessary healthcare expenditures.

Equally important is the emphasis on open and transparent communication between all parties involved. Regular interdisciplinary meetings, collaborative rounds, and integrated electronic health records foster a culture of teamwork and shared accountability. Through these mechanisms, Case Managers can keep everyone informed about changes in a patient's condition, progress toward goals, and any adjustments needed to the care plan. This collaborative approach not only streamlines transitions of care, such as from hospital to home or rehabilitation, but also enhances patient satisfaction by ensuring that their needs and preferences are consistently respected.

Ultimately, Case Management's integration across provider and payor sectors strengthens the entire healthcare delivery system. By bridging gaps between clinical care, insurance regulations, and community resources, Case Managers help create a seamless continuum that prioritizes both quality and efficiency. Their multifaceted role is essential in navigating today's complex healthcare environment, ensuring that all patients—regardless of their circumstances—receive compassionate, coordinated, and cost-effective care.

The integration of Case Management within the healthcare setting is a dynamic and crucial component of contemporary healthcare delivery. As we move forward, it is essential to continue to emphasize the collaborative nature of Case Management, the importance of communication and teamwork, and the effective utilization of technology and data. By doing so, we can ensure that the complex needs of patients are met with efficiency and compassion, leading to a more robust and effective healthcare system that prioritizes the well-being of every individual it serves. This ongoing transformation is not merely an operational necessity; it is a fundamental commitment to enhancing the quality of care and improving the health of our communities as a whole.

1.3 Case Management Models in Healthcare

In the realm of healthcare, effective case management is vital for ensuring that patients receive optimal care throughout their treatment journey. Case management plays a crucial role in coordinating various services, facilitating communication between healthcare providers, and guiding patients to navigate their healthcare experience. Various case management models exist, each designed to meet specific facility needs and address diverse patient demands. These models can range from disease-specific management to more holistic approaches that integrate social determinants of health. Understanding the strengths and limitations of these models is crucial in selecting the most appropriate approach for a given healthcare setting.

Additionally, the successful implementation of a chosen model can lead to improved patient outcomes, reduced hospital readmissions, and achieve higher levels of patient satisfaction. As healthcare continues to evolve, particularly with the rise of technology and personalized medicine, the role of case management will likely become even more significant, adapting to new challenges and opportunities in patient care. Therefore, healthcare professionals must remain informed about the latest trends and best practices in case management to ensure that they can provide the highest quality of care for their patients.

1.4 Collaborative Roles of Nurses and Social Workers

Many healthcare facilities utilize a combination of nurses and social workers to fulfill essential case management roles. This interdisciplinary approach is increasingly recognized as a method to enhance patient care by addressing both medical and psychosocial needs. Nurses are primarily responsible for the clinical assessment and management of health conditions, providing direct care and monitoring patients' medical needs. They ensure that patients receive the appropriate interventions and treatments while advocating for their overall health and well-being.

On the other hand, social workers play a crucial role in addressing the social determinants of health, which encompass a range of factors such as socioeconomic status, education, neighborhood, and social support networks. These factors significantly influence an individual's health outcomes and access to care. Social workers are trained to evaluate and assist patients in navigating challenges they might face outside of the clinical setting, such as obtaining financial assistance, housing resources, or mental health support. By doing so, they help create a comprehensive support system that addresses the multifaceted needs of patients.

However, this collaborative approach can also pose challenges. For instance, nursing professionals may lack the specialized skills and training to effectively address the social determinants of health that social workers are expertly equipped to handle. Conversely, social workers might not have the clinical knowledge necessary for managing complex medical conditions, which can lead to gaps in care if not properly coordinated.

To maximize the effectiveness of case management, it is essential to leverage each professional's expertise in accordance with their training and licensure. This means fostering an environment of mutual respect and open communication, where both nurses and social workers can share insights and collaborate on care plans. Regular interdisciplinary meetings can facilitate this collaboration, allowing team members to discuss patient cases, share knowledge, and develop joint strategies that prioritize patient outcomes and well-being. By recognizing and valuing the distinct roles of nurses and social workers, healthcare facilities can create a more integrated care approach, ultimately leading to improved health outcomes for the patient population they serve.

1.5 The Dyad Model: Balancing Utilization Review and Discharge Planning

One prevalent model of case management in the healthcare industry is known as the Dyad Model. In this framework, a single case manager is tasked with the dual responsibilities of Utilization Review and Discharge Planning. This approach is particularly well-suited for smaller healthcare facilities that experience a lower patient census. By integrating these two functions under one individual, the Dyad Model helps to manage workforce expenses more effectively while fostering a deeper understanding of each patient's unique care trajectory and needs. However, as healthcare systems evolve and the demand for services increases, the dynamic of this model can shift dramatically, particularly in larger facilities or environments with higher patient turnover.

As the case manager's focus becomes heavily weighted toward discharge planning, often due to pressures to expedite patient movement, there may be a significant decline in essential care coordination. This reduced emphasis on comprehensive resource utilization can have far-reaching consequences. Specifically, it can lead to increased instances of insurance claim denials, wherein payors do not receive timely or complete information necessary for processing claims. The outcome of these administrative challenges can ultimately result in avoidable delays in patient care and unnecessarily prolonged hospital stays. These complications not only impact operational efficiency but also diminish the overall quality of patient experience and healthcare delivery. Balancing these responsibilities is crucial for optimizing outcomes in this complex healthcare landscape.

1.6 The Triad Model: Enhancing Collaboration and Care Quality

In contrast to traditional care management approaches, the Triad Model advocates a clearer division of responsibilities, with separate, specialized teams handling Utilization Review and Case Management. This innovative structure is particularly beneficial in larger healthcare facilities, where the complexity and volume of patient cases can strain resources and time. By establishing this distinct separation of duties, the Triad Model accommodates the increased demands for time and attention that both functions require, facilitating a more organized workflow.

By implementing the Triad Model, case managers are empowered to dedicate the necessary time to collaborate effectively with the multidisciplinary care team, which may include physicians, nurses, social workers, and other allied health professionals. This collaboration ensures comprehensive patient care while also facilitating timely transitions between different levels of care, whether that involves moving a patient from the emergency room to an inpatient setting or ensuring a smooth discharge to home health services.

Concurrently, the staff dedicated to Utilization Review can focus entirely on liaising with payors, acquiring necessary authorizations, and promptly addressing any potential denials that may arise during the care process. By concentrating their efforts, these team members can navigate the often-complex landscape of insurance requirements more efficiently, reducing the likelihood of delays in patient care.

Although the increased need for staffing may raise operational costs in the short term, the resulting improvements in patient outcomes and overall care quality can easily justify this investment. Ultimately, the Triad Model not only enhances the efficiency of care delivery but also fosters a collaborative environment that prioritizes patient well-being, ensuring that each patient receives the personalized attention and support they need throughout their healthcare journey. This comprehensive approach can lead to higher patient satisfaction rates and better health outcomes, solidifying the value of the Triad Model in modern healthcare settings.

1.7 Role of Non-Licensed Staff

Regardless of the model employed, many healthcare facilities actively engage non-licensed personnel to assist case managers, nurses, and social workers in managing various administrative and clerical tasks. These non-licensed staff members contribute significantly by undertaking responsibilities such as managing phone calls, obtaining patient signatures, and facilitating documentation processes. By handling these essential tasks, they play a vital role in enhancing workforce efficiency and overall productivity within healthcare teams.

Their contributions allow licensed professionals to concentrate more fully on direct patient care and complex decision-making, ultimately leading to improved patient outcomes. When licensed staff can focus on what they do best, they are better equipped to address patient needs, provide high-quality care, and make informed clinical decisions.

The non-licensed personnel can also serve as a bridge between patients and licensed staff, improving communication and ensuring that patient concerns are promptly addressed. This collaborative approach fosters a more supportive healthcare environment where everyone's strengths are utilized effectively. In conclusion, selecting the right case management model is crucial for optimizing patient care, particularly in complex healthcare environments. By understanding each model's unique characteristics and effectively utilizing interdisciplinary teams, healthcare facilities can enhance their service delivery, streamline processes, and ultimately improve patient outcomes.

2 Regulations and Compliance Impacting Case Management

Learning Objectives

1. **Understand Key Regulations:** Gain a comprehensive understanding of the regulations imposed by the Centers for Medicare & Medicaid Services (CMS) and the Conditions of Participation as they relate to case management.
2. **Familiarity with Accreditation Standards**: Develop knowledge of how compliance with these regulations impacts accreditation surveys and overall care quality, preparing case managers to meet organizational standards.
3. **Continuous Education:** Recognize the importance of ongoing education regarding evolving regulations to ensure that case managers remain compliant and informed about changes that may affect patient care.
4. **Impact on Patient Outcomes:** Analyze how a thorough understanding of regulatory requirements enhances patient outcomes and service delivery, emphasizing the role of case managers in quality improvement.
5. **Advocacy and Navigation:** Empower case managers to effectively navigate challenges within the healthcare system, enabling them to advocate for patients while promoting accountability and quality in care delivery.

The Centers for Medicare & Medicaid Services (CMS) and the Conditions of Participation impose significant regulations on our profession, making it essential for Case Managers to possess a thorough understanding of these guidelines. Familiarity with the specific areas governed by these regulations is crucial, as they directly impact accreditation surveys and the overall quality of care provided.

Case Managers must continually educate themselves on the evolving regulations to ensure compliance and enhance patient outcomes. This knowledge not only strengthens

S. Garceau, *Interdisciplinary Case Management: A Nursing Practice Approach*,
https://doi.org/10.1007/978-3-032-20960-3_2

their professional practice but also supports the organization in meeting accreditation standards, ultimately leading to improved service delivery and patient satisfaction. Understanding these regulatory requirements empowers Case Managers to navigate challenges effectively, advocate for patients, and contribute to a system that prioritizes quality and accountability in healthcare.

2.1 Conditions of Participation

Utilization Review

Utilization Review (UR) is a critical component of the Case Management or Utilization Management staff responsibilities, ensuring that all cases are thoroughly screened for medical necessity. This process involves applying standardized criteria to evaluate whether the care provided aligns with established guidelines and is necessary for the patient's health outcome. The initial reviews can take place before admission or during the admission process and continue throughout the patient's stay in the facility. Additionally, retrospective reviews can be conducted after the patient has been discharged to ensure that all medical requirements were met during their hospitalization (Fig. 2.1).

A key aspect of reviewing cases for Medicare procedures includes determining if the procedure is listed on the Centers for Medicare & Medicaid Services (CMS) inpatient-only (IPO) list. For any procedure categorized as inpatient-only, it is essential that the procedure is performed in a hospital setting and that an inpatient order is documented in the patient's chart before both the procedure and the patient's discharge. However, even if a procedure does not appear on the IPO list, it is still crucial to assess the documentation of medical necessity since there can be valid reasons for performing certain procedures in an inpatient environment.

It is important to note that CMS does not maintain an outpatient-only list, meaning medical necessity remains a pivotal factor for all procedures, independently of their classification.

Discharge Planning and Conflict of Interest

As mandated by CMS, discharge planning must be initiated with a screening conducted within 24 h of the patient's admission. The Case Manager plays a crucial role in this process. If the Case Manager identifies potential risks to the patient, if the patient or their family requests an evaluation, or if facility staff raise concerns, it becomes essential for the Case Manager to perform a thorough evaluation. This evaluation should address potential risks, assess social determinants of health that could affect patient outcomes, and initiate measures to mitigate any identified issues. For example, this could involve providing resources or referrals for the patient or their support system to access independently.

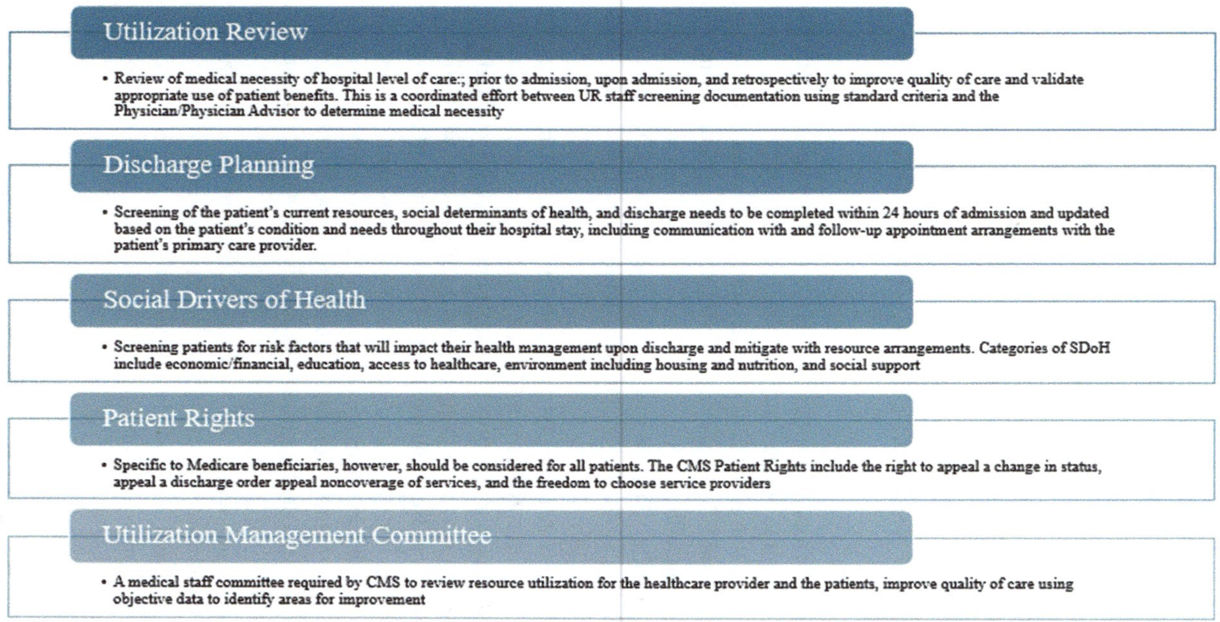

Fig. 2.1 Highlights the key Conditions of Participation including a description for each element. Created by the author

Effective discharge planning also requires careful communication and coordination of post-discharge follow-up appointments with the patient's primary care provider. This ensures continuity of care as the patient transitions back to the community and begins receiving outpatient services.

Transparency is paramount in the discharge planning process. It is essential to keep the patient or their representative informed about any potential conflicts of interest that may arise. A conflict of interest occurs when the healthcare facility or provider has a financial stake in a post-discharge service that the patient may use. Regulations, such as the Stark Law, specifically address these issues. Violations of Stark Law could lead to significant ramifications, including denial of payment, civil penalties, or exclusion from participation in Medicare and Medicaid programs (Fig. 2.2).

Social Drivers of Health (SDoH) and Health-Related Social Needs (HRSN)

The term "Social Drives of Health" (SDOH), sometimes called Social Determinants of Health, refers to the various social conditions in which people are born, grow, live, work, and age that significantly impact their health outcomes. According to the Centers for Medicare & Medicaid Services (CMS), SDOH/HRSN encompass a wide range of factors, including:

Economic Stability: This includes employment, income, expenses, and financial support, all of which influence individuals' ability to access healthcare services and maintain overall health.

Education Access and Quality: Education plays a critical role in health literacy and access to health information, influencing lifestyle choices and health behaviors.

Healthcare Access and Quality: This factor considers the availability of healthcare services, health insurance coverage, and the quality of care received.

Neighborhood and Built Environment: The conditions of a person's living environment, including housing quality, access to nutritious food, public transportation, and safe areas for physical activity, significantly affect health.

Social and Community Context: This includes the relationships and networks individuals have within their community, which can provide social support and impact mental well-being.

Understanding and addressing these social determinants is vital for improving overall public health and reducing health disparities among different populations. By incorporating SDOH/HRSN into healthcare policy and practice, organizations like CMS aim to create more equitable health outcomes and enhance the effectiveness of health programs.

Patient Rights (as Applies to Case Management Roles)

The Conditions of Participation (CoPs) are a set of federal regulations that healthcare providers must comply with in order to participate in Medicare and Medicaid

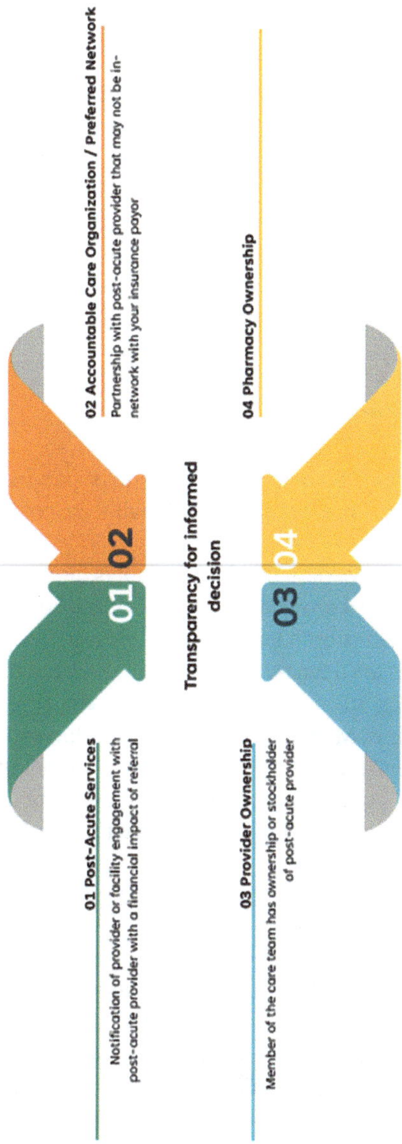

Fig. 2.2 Describes the areas in healthcare that must be disclosed to patients in order to provide transparency in relationship between providers. Created by the author

programs. These regulations establish standards for the quality and safety of patient care, ensuring that healthcare organizations meet certain requirements in areas such as patient rights, staffing, and infection control.

Patients are encouraged to actively participate in developing and implementing their care plans. This collaborative approach fosters stronger relationships between the patient and healthcare professionals, ensuring the patient's voice is heard with their values and preferences respected

Key aspects of the Conditions of Participation include requirements for patient treatment, protection of patient rights, continuous quality improvement, and requirements for clinical records and patient care policies. Compliance with these standards is crucial for providers to receive federal funding and maintain their licensure. One specific section, such as § 482.13, addresses the rights of patients, emphasizing the importance of respecting and protecting these rights throughout the care process.

Overall, the CoPs aim to enhance the quality of care delivered to patients in healthcare facilities while ensuring their safety and rights are upheld.

Choice of Providers (Freedom of Choice)

Patients have the inherent right to choose from a range of providers that are part of their insurance plan. This empowers them to select healthcare professionals who best align with their needs and preferences.

For beneficiaries of Medicare and Medicaid, this right is further enhanced, allowing them to choose from any qualified provider, even those outside the confines of specific networks. This flexibility ensures broader access to necessary medical care.

The right to choose applies to all types of healthcare providers, including physicians, hospitals, and institutions that offer post-acute care services.

The Centers for Medicare & Medicaid Services (CMS) has established discharge planning requirements. These regulations assist patients in making informed decisions about their options for post-acute care providers, ensuring they have access to comprehensive data on the quality of care and resource utilization.

Informed Decisions About Care

Patients possess the right to make informed decisions regarding their healthcare. This includes receiving comprehensive information about their health status, available treatment options, and the potential risks and benefits associated with each option.

Patients are encouraged to actively participate in the development and implementation of their individual care plans. This collaborative approach enhances patient engagement and promotes shared decision-making between patients and healthcare professionals.

The right to request or refuse treatment is central to patient autonomy, provided that such requests align with medical appropriateness and do not infringe upon other established patient rights.

Informed consent is the cornerstone of ethical medical practice, ensuring that treatment decisions are made transparently and with the patient's values and preferences in mind.

Advance Directives

Patients have the right to create advanced directives, including living wills and medical power of attorney, which express their healthcare preferences in situations where they may be unable to communicate their wishes.

It is the responsibility of hospital staff and healthcare practitioners to honor these directives in accordance with federal regulations. This respect for patient autonomy ensures that individual values and desires are upheld even when patients cannot advocate for themselves.

Family Notification

Patients are entitled to have a family member or representative of their choice, along with their personal physician, notified promptly following their admission to a healthcare facility. This inclusion fosters a support system during what can be a stressful time for patients.

Privacy and Safety

Patients have the right to privacy and safety throughout their care experience, ensuring that their dignity is preserved.

They must be protected from any form of abuse or harassment during their treatment. Regulations like the Health Insurance Portability and Accountability Act (HIPAA) safeguard the confidentiality of patient records and personal health information.

Access to Records

Patients have the right to access their medical records, including any records that are kept in electronic format. This transparency promotes patient empowerment and engagement in their health journey.

Patients are entitled to have their medical information secure, free from unnecessary exposure or mishandling.

Freedom from Abuse

Patients maintain the unequivocal right to be free from any form of physical or mental abuse, as well as corporal punishment. This right is foundational to fostering a safe and respectful healthcare environment.

Right to Appeal

Appeals for Changes in Patient Status

Patients have the right to appeal classifications related to their care status, including the reclassification from inpatient to outpatient observation. This right ensures that patients can contest and seek clarification regarding their treatment designations, which can significantly affect their care and billing processes.

Appeal of Discharge

Under CMS guidelines, Medicare beneficiaries have the right to appeal a hospital discharge decision if they believe it's not medically appropriate. They can request an expedited review before leaving the hospital by filing a claim with the Beneficiary and Family Centered Care—Quality Improvement Organization (BFCC-QIO) or QIO. This appeal process allows beneficiaries to challenge a hospital's decision to reclassify them from inpatient to outpatient observation, potentially denying coverage for their hospital stay

Appeal of Noncoverage

As a Medicare or Medicare Advantage beneficiary, patients have the right to appeal a determination of noncoverage for services, including outpatient services, coverage of services during a hospital admission, and the end of coverage for services.

These rights underscore the commitment to uphold patient dignity, autonomy, and well-being in all healthcare interactions, fostering an environment that respects individual choices and promotes patient-centered care.

Utilization Management Committee (UMC)

The Utilization Management Committee is the only committee mandated by CMS. It is a Medical Staff committee that reviews the utilization of resources for both the facility and the use of patient benefits. The committee identifies quality improvement opportunities, assists facility leadership in prioritizing quality care and monitoring processes. UMC reports through to the facility Board of Directors for additional recommendations and provides accountability.

Overall, these rules and processes are designed to enhance patient care, ensure proper documentation, and provide beneficiaries with the necessary information to navigate their healthcare effectively. By adhering to these guidelines, healthcare providers can ensure that patients receive the appropriate care while also being kept informed of their rights and responsibilities within the Medicare system.

2.2 CMS Forms and Requirements

Two Midnight Rule (2MN)

To reduce inpatient admission errors, in fiscal year 2014, CMS implemented the Two-Midnight Rule. CMS generally considers it inappropriate to receive payment under the inpatient prospective payment system for stays not expected to span at least two midnights.

The requirements include: Inpatient services are considered appropriate if the physician expects the patient to require medically necessary hospital care spanning at least two midnights.

Inpatient services are also appropriate if the physician is providing a service listed as "inpatient only" by Medicare; even if the physician expects the care to be less than two midnights, inpatient services may still be warranted based on their professional judgment; the two-Midnight Rule allows hospitals to account for total hospital time (including outpatient time directly proceeding the inpatient admission) when determining if an inpatient admission order should be written based on the expectation that the beneficiary will stay in the hospital for two or more midnights receiving medically necessary care.

As of January 2024, the Centers for Medicare & Medicaid Services (CMS) has implemented the Two Midnight Rule (2MN) for Medicare Advantage Plans (MA). This regulation stipulates that when a patient has been in the hospital for one midnight (1MN) and there is a projected need for hospital care extending to a second midnight (2MN), with appropriate and clear documentation from the attending healthcare provider, it is generally reasonable to transition the patient's status to an inpatient admission. This rule is designed to ensure that patients who genuinely require further hospital care are not unduly classified as outpatient, thus allowing them to access the benefits and coverage associated with inpatient status.

As with all rules, there are exceptions, inclusions, and exemptions to the Two-Midnight Rule (Fig. 2.3).

Condition Code 44 (Including Medicare Outpatient Observation Notice and Medicare Change in Status Notification)

For traditional Medicare, a specific protocol must be followed when a patient's hospital admission is considered for downgrade from inpatient to either outpatient or outpatient with observation status. This process mandates a comprehensive review by a second physician who must concur with the attending physician's assessment that a downgrade is warranted. This change must be thoroughly documented in the

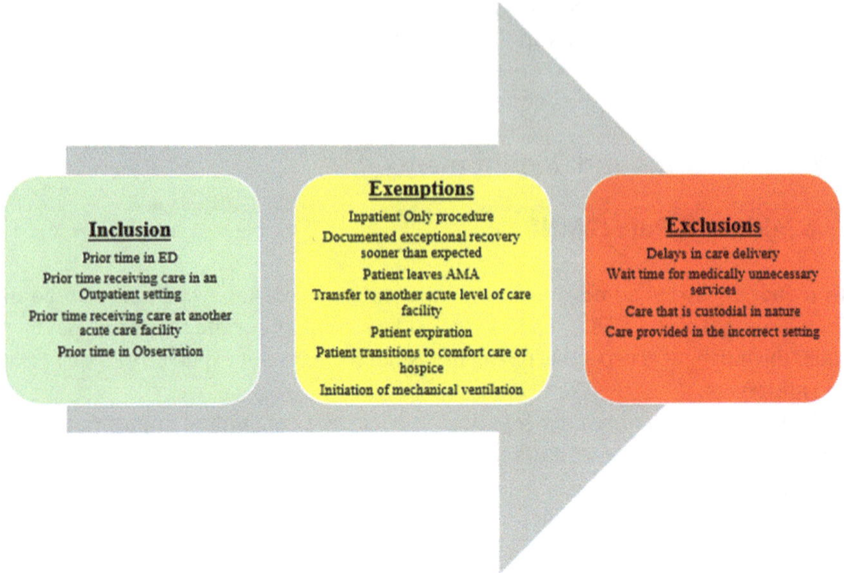

Fig. 2.3 CMS provides clear guidelines to determine care included, excluded and exemptions to the 2-Midnight Rule. Created by the author

patient's medical record. It is critical to formally notify the patient in writing about this adjustment in status, as it has significant implications for their out-of-pocket expenses. This notification is achieved through the issuance of the Medicare Outpatient Observation Notice (MOON), which is also provided to all Medicare beneficiaries who are placed directly into observation status. Ensuring that patients understand their financial responsibilities and healthcare status is a key component of this process.

Condition Code 44 (CC44) is specific to traditional Medicare beneficiaries and addresses cases in which an inpatient admission was changed to an outpatient admission. The billing code "44" must be placed on outpatient claims only when the physician ordered inpatient services, but upon internal review performed before the claim was initially submitted, the hospital determined the services did not meet its inpatient criteria. Prior to the condition code being placed on the bill, there are required steps that must occur prior to the patient's discharge. First, the attending provider must concur with the determination to downgrade the patient's level of care; if the provider does not concur with the opportunity to present the case to the UM Committee or QIO prior to the final determination, if the outcome of this discussion is to downgrade the patient, the provider will enter the new level of care order to include the reason for the downgrade. The final step is key to meeting the CMS requirement. The patient and/or representative must be provided with the Medicare Change in Status Notice (MCSN) and the Medicare Outpatient Observation Notice (MOON). The MCSN allows the patient to initiate their right to appeal the change in status, while the MOON provides notification of the status, which includes the financial impact for the patient. Both forms should be signed, with a copy included in the patient's medical record. Once the steps outlined have been completed and documented by the Case Management staff, the billing department can place the code on the claim.

There is one consideration that must be reviewed prior to proceeding with a level of care downgrade. Review of the record for services that support the Medicare Two-Midnight Rule is included in the Occurrence Span Code 72, another billing code that is added to the claim either concurrently or retrospectively. These services include observation-level care, two or more days of admission, and prior services provided in an outpatient setting, such as the Emergency Department or in a procedural area.

Important Message from Medicare (IMM)

Upon admission to a hospital, all Medicare beneficiaries receive the Important Message from Medicare (IMM). This essential document is intended to inform patients of their rights regarding hospitalization, particularly the right to appeal a discharge order. It clearly outlines the steps that patients need to take if they decide to contest their discharge. Should a patient choose to appeal, the hospital is obligated to provide additional documentation that offers further details and guidance, aiding the patient in making an informed decision regarding their appeal. The IMM serves to empower beneficiaries, ensuring they are aware of and can exercise their rights throughout their care journey.

The Important Message from Medicare (IM) is a standard notice that must be delivered to all Medicare and Managed Medicare (MA) beneficiaries order for Inpatient. As with all CMS forms, the IMM form is an Office of Management and Budget (OMB) approved form and **cannot** be altered from its original form, including font and format. Hospital information must be added to the appropriate fields.

The timeframe for the delivery of the form is clearly spelled out in the Condition of Participation (CoP) **§482.13(a)(1):** At the time of admission, within 48 h prior to discharge (if discharge is within 48 h of admission, you do not need an additional IMM), but no less than 4 h prior to discharge.

Recertification and Extended Stay Review

For Medicare beneficiaries whose hospital stays extend beyond 20 days, documentation of a recertification, affirming the medical necessity for continued hospitalization, is required to be entered into the patient's medical record. For behavioral health admissions, this requirement extends to 30 days. The recertification process is crucial for maintaining oversight of patient care and resources. It involves a thorough review of each extended stay case by the hospital's Utilization Management Committee, which evaluates the appropriateness of ongoing inpatient care. This committee plays a vital role in ensuring that hospitals are delivering high-quality care while maintaining compliance with Medicare regulations.

Recertification requirements have a variation based on the setting. Acute care hospitals have the requirement of an inpatient level of care necessity initial certification within 24 h of admission and then recertification at day 20 of the admission followed by every 7 days after that time. This includes review of the case by the UM Committee physicians as a secondary review of the case and supporting medical necessity.

Behavioral health requires the initial certification within 12 days of hospitalization, upon day 30 and every 7 days after that point. Again, this includes review by the UM Committee physicians.

There are other regulatory and compliance areas that are not covered in the Conditions of Participation, which we will now discuss.

Hospital Issued Notice of Noncoverage (HINN)

There are four different HINN forms used for Medicare and Medicare Advantage (MA) beneficiaries within the acute care hospital (Fig. 2.4).

Several facilities across the country have opted to create similar forms for use with patients who are not covered by Medicare or an MA plan.

There are also forms specific to outpatient services, which providers and/or plans are required to provide patients with a new process in place, allowing the patient to appeal the non-coverage.

Other payors also have specific required forms that Case Management should be aware of and, as part of the role of reviewing the patient record, ensure that the form is completed and has been submitted in a timely manner.

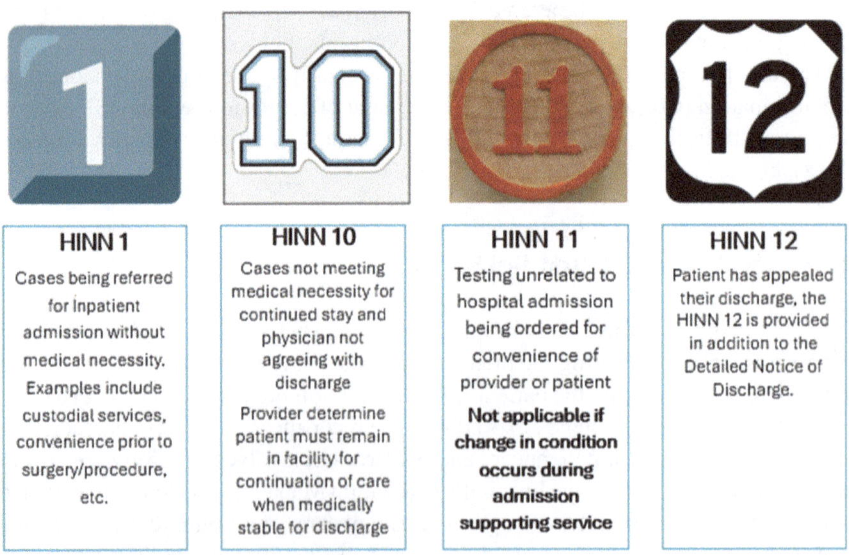

Fig. 2.4 Provides a high-level description of the different CMS Hospital Issued Notices of Noncoverage forms. Created by the author

2.3 Patient Protection and Complaint Investigation

Office of the Inspector General (OIG)

The Office of the Inspector General (OIG) plays a crucial role in overseeing the operations and integrity of the Department of Health and Human Services (HHS). Through a comprehensive approach that combines data analytics and modeling, alongside criminal, civil, and administrative investigations, the OIG is dedicated to safeguarding patient rights and ensuring their safety within the healthcare system.

The OIG collaborates closely with various stakeholders, including HHS staff, operating divisions, the Department of Justice, and other executive branch agencies. This multi-faceted cooperation extends to Congress, state authorities, and representatives from the private sector. The goal of these partnerships is to drive systemic improvements in the healthcare landscape, enhance compliance with regulations, enforce necessary actions against misconduct, and recover funds that have been misappropriated. A significant part of the OIG's mission involves the proactive identification and prevention of fraud, waste, and abuse in healthcare services.

Beneficiary and Family Centered Care – Quality Improvement Organization (BFCC-QIO)

Spearheaded by the Centers for Medicare & Medicaid Services (CMS), the Quality Improvement Organization (QIO) Program represents one of the largest federal initiatives aimed at enhancing healthcare quality for Medicare beneficiaries. Established in 1982 under Title XI of the Social Security Act, the QIO Program is a vital component of HHS's strategy to promote equitable access to high-quality, affordable healthcare services.

The core functions of the QIO Program are multifaceted and include:

Data-Driven Quality Improvement: Utilizing data analysis to monitor and track improvements in healthcare quality at the local level, ensuring that care delivery meets established standards.

Protection of the Medicare System: Ensuring that Medicare funds are disbursed only for services and goods that are deemed reasonable and necessary and that these services are delivered in the most appropriate settings.

Beneficiary Advocacy: Addressing beneficiary complaints effectively and implementing provider-based appeals, as well as overseeing compliance with regulations such as the Emergency Medical Treatment and Labor Act (EMTALA).

Through these initiatives, the QIO Program works tirelessly to enhance patient experiences and outcomes. It promotes behavioral health improvements, reduces opioid misuse, enhances chronic disease management, and strengthens care coordination and transition of care processes. Additionally, the program focuses on increasing immunization rates, bolstering patient safety standards, and improving infection control measures across healthcare settings.

In the United States, there are two primary Quality Improvement Organizations: Acentra Health and Livanta. Each of these organizations is responsible for specific states, acting as the main point of contact for patients who wish to voice concerns or exercise their right to appeal decisions regarding their care. By bridging the gap between beneficiaries and healthcare providers, the QIO plays a pivotal role in maintaining high-quality standards and ensuring that patient needs are met consistently.

2.4 Facility Accreditation

Auditing/Survey Agencies

The oversight of compliance with the Centers for Medicare & Medicaid Services (CMS) requirements is primarily carried out by two leading survey agencies: The Joint Commission (TJC) and Det Norske Veritas (DNV). These organizations play a crucial role in monitoring healthcare facilities to ensure they meet the stringent standards set forth by CMS, particularly concerning critical areas like Utilization Review as outlined in §482.30 and Discharge Planning in §482.43.

The primary objective of TJC and DNV is to facilitate a comprehensive approach to patient safety and care quality. By conducting thorough evaluations, these agencies ensure that healthcare facilities not only adhere to regulatory requirements but also implement best practices that enhance patient outcomes.

In their assessments, the surveyors delve into various aspects of healthcare delivery, including the effectiveness of utilization review processes that help manage patient care efficiently and responsibly. They also examine discharge planning protocols to ensure that patients transition safely out of care settings, reducing the likelihood of readmission and promoting continuity of care.

Through their diligent oversight, TJC and DNV contribute to fostering a culture of safety and quality in healthcare, enabling facilities to deliver the highest level of patient-centered care while maintaining compliance with federal regulations (Fig. 2.5).

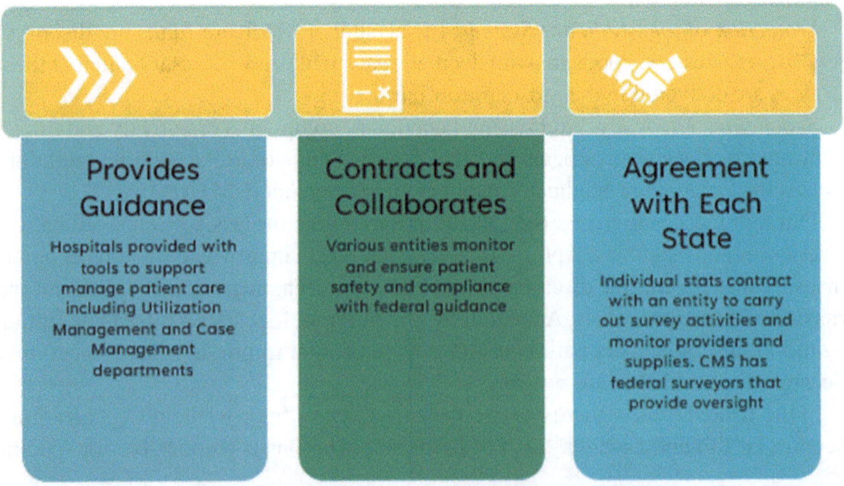

Fig. 2.5 Illustrates the key process supported by auditing and survey agencies. Created by the author

TJC and DNV, along with other accrediting agencies, evaluate hospitals to ensure compliance with CMS Conditions of Participation and quality care standards. These surveys aim to enhance patient safety, improve care quality, and identify areas needing improvement. Successful accreditation boosts the facility's reputation and fosters trust and satisfaction among staff, providers, and the community.

2.5 Case Studies

Two-Midnight Rule

A 79-year-old Medicare beneficiary presents with a Congestive Heart Failure (CHF) exacerbation. Oxygen saturations are 90% on home oxygen, with a congested cough, and the chest X-ray supports fluid overload. The patient also has severe Chronic Obstructive Pulmonary Disease (COPD) requiring home oxygen at 2 L per nasal canula, and arthritis. The Primary Care Provider's office documents state the patient was in the hospital for 6 days due to pulmonary problems during the last admission 2 months ago. Orders for oxygen, telemetry, pulse oximetry, respiratory nebulizer treatments scheduled and as needed, and intravenous diuresis. Documentation from the attending states that due to the patient's advanced age, history of slow and complicated recovery recently, and frequent assessment requirements, the expected length of stay will be greater than two midnights.

Due to the high-risk patient with reasons to expect a longer stay with a well-documented treatment plan supporting hospital-level care, an Inpatient order is placed.

Is an inpatient admission appropriate for this Medicare beneficiary?

Yes, this case demonstrates requirements to meet the CMS two-midnight rule: duration of stay and medical necessity for care.

Conflict of Interest

A hospital Case Manager is asked to meet with a patient and family to discuss discharge needs, which include home health nursing and therapy needs. The Case Manager's significant other is a physical therapist for a local home health agency. The Case Manager provides the patient with a list of available home health agencies and includes a recommendation for a "well-respected agency" that happens to be the one where the significant other is employed, without divulging that there is a potential benefit to the Case Manager if that agency is selected.

Would this be a conflict of interest?

Yes, per the law, without disclosure to the patient and family *and* the recommendation this is a clear conflict of interest due to the financial benefit to the Case Manager (Conditions for Coverage (CfCs) & Conditions of Participation (CoPs) | CMS 2026; Notices and Forms | CMS 2026).

References

Conditions for Coverage (CfCs) & Conditions of Participation (CoPs) | CMS (2026). Accessed 1 Mar 2025
Notices and Forms | CMS (2026). Accessed 1 Mar 2025

3 Case Management Settings

Learning Objectives

1. **Understand the Role of Case Managers:** Identify the responsibilities and functions of Case Managers across various healthcare settings, emphasizing their importance in enhancing patient care.
2. **Recognize the Person-Centered Approach:** Explain the significance of a person-centered approach in Case Management, focusing on the establishment of trust and effective communication between Case Managers and patients.
3. **Develop Comprehensive Care Plans:** Learn how to create comprehensive care plans that address individual patient needs, incorporating necessary interventions, resources, and support systems.
4. **Facilitate Seamless Care Transitions:** Describe the strategies Case Managers use to ensure smooth transitions for patients, particularly during the shift from acute care to outpatient settings, and the importance of reducing barriers to access.
5. **Utilize Technology in Case Management:** Examine the impact of technology, including Electronic Health Records (EHRs) and telehealth, on Case Management practices and patient tracking, as well as how data analytics can improve patient outcomes.
6. **Engage Patients Effectively:** Explore techniques such as motivational interviewing and active listening that Case Managers can use to better engage with patients and understand their unique health needs.
7. **Evaluate Outcomes and Trends:** Analyze how Case Managers can leverage data to monitor patient progress and trends that affect care, enabling proactive interventions.

S. Garceau, *Interdisciplinary Case Management: A Nursing Practice Approach*,
https://doi.org/10.1007/978-3-032-20960-3_3

As healthcare continues to evolve with an increasing reliance on technology and innovative practices, the role of the Case Manager has grown in both significance and complexity. Case Managers are integral members of care teams across numerous healthcare settings, tasked with shaping the future of patient care and enhancing communication throughout the continuum of care. Their work plays a pivotal role in improving patient outcomes and overall quality of life.

With the expanding role of Case Managers, it's essential to understand not only their responsibilities but also the systems in which they operate. They ensure patients can navigate the often overwhelming healthcare landscape, reducing barriers to access and facilitating essential services tailored to individual needs.

3.1 The Foundation of Case Management

At the core of effective Case Management is the understanding that each patient is unique. This person-centered approach affirms the necessity of establishing strong relationships between Case Managers and patients. These relationships are built on trust, communication, and empathy. Case Managers utilize a variety of strategies, including motivational interviewing techniques and active listening, to ascertain a patient's needs fully.

Once patients are assessed, Case Managers develop comprehensive care plans that outline the necessary interventions, resources, and support systems. This plan serves not only as a guide for the patient but also as a communication tool for all parties involved in the patient's care. The collaborative approach is particularly essential in ensuring seamless care transitions, especially when moving from acute to outpatient settings. This transition can often be a vulnerable time for patients, and proactive Case Management serves to alleviate some of this stress.

3.2 The Role of Technology

The influx of technology in healthcare has transformed Case Management. Electronic Health Records (EHRs) and data analytics tools now assist Case Managers in tracking patient progress and identifying trends that may affect care. For example, data collected through EHRs can help Case Managers identify patients who frequently visit emergency departments. With this information, they can engage with these patients more intensively, providing them with the knowledge and resources needed to manage their health better in the community.

Telehealth has also become an essential part of Case Management. With the rise of remote consultation services, Case Managers can reach a broader patient population, especially those in rural or underserved areas. They can facilitate virtual appointments, ensuring that patients still have access to their healthcare providers without the need for extensive travel or wait times. This flexible model not only improves access to care but also empowers patients to take an active role in managing their health.

3.3 Coordination Across Healthcare Settings

Case Managers are typically employed in acute care settings such as Short-Term Acute Care Hospitals (STACH), Long-Term Acute Care Hospitals (LTACH), Skilled Nursing Facilities (SNF), Acute Inpatient Rehabilitation Facilities (IRF/ARF), and Inpatient Behavioral Health Hospitals (BH). Each of these environments presents its own challenges and necessitates that Case Managers possess a robust understanding of operational processes and protocols.

In acute care settings, the focus is often on immediate patient needs—addressing acute conditions, pain management, and coordinating post-discharge care. Case Managers in these environments must work diligently to prepare patients for a safe transition back to their homes or to other settings, which may include rehabilitation facilities or skilled nursing. The acute care setting typically requires quick thinking and immediate coordination of services, emphasizing the need for strong organizational and communication skills.

However, the scope of Case Management extends far into outpatient settings. Here, Case Managers focus on connecting identified patients with resources that significantly enhance their overall health and well-being. For outpatients, the services they may require can include financial assistance, housing support, meal programs, employment search services, and child or elder care. As healthcare systems increasingly emphasize preventative care, the work of Case Managers in outpatient settings plays a crucial role in reducing hospital readmissions and ensuring patients maintain their health over time.

Case Managers are also an integral part of the payor team. The payor CM team assists with the Utilization Review and authorization process as well as the transition of patients from the acute care setting, post-acute provider service, back to the community. Payor CM teams also assist patients in identifying programs available to support optimal health maintenance.

3.4 Collaboration with Payors

As previously discussed, Case Management involves engagement at the insurance provider level, where Case Managers and Utilization Review specialists work seamlessly to facilitate appropriate coverage for payor beneficiaries. This collaboration ensures that patients receive the services they need when required. Case Managers often serve as the bridge between patients and payors, helping to demystify insurance processes and enabling patients to understand their benefits and coverages.

This role was already significant prior to recent healthcare reforms, but its importance has only intensified. With policies aimed at reducing costs and improving efficiency, understanding the intricacies of insurance coverage is essential for Case Managers. They must be well-versed in navigating denials, prior authorizations, and appeals processes within various insurance plans. By doing this, Case Managers not only provide immediate support to their patients but also advocate for system-wide improvements that promote patient care continuity.

3.5 Care Navigation and the Role of the Navigation Nurse or Social Worker

As healthcare advances and patient healthcare needs become more important, the role of the Navigator within health care has emerged. This role can be surgical or medical focus in scope, but offers patients an expert in understanding the plan and trajectory of care.

Within the surgical arena, the Navigator is integrated into the patients care team from the initial visit to the surgeon's office. The Navigator helps with scheduling the required prerequisite treatments or screenings are completed ensuring that all necessary documentation is accurately prepared and submitted to the payor when required. Acting as both advocate and educator, the Navigator guides patients and their support networks through the expected course of care, outlining recovery needs specific to each planned procedure. This proactive approach empowers patients and families to fully comprehend the discharge process and, when applicable, to make informed choices about post-procedure care. Clear, consistent communication between the Navigator, the patient, and providers helps facilitate smooth transitions and alleviates concerns, promoting a supportive and informed healthcare experience.

For patients living with chronic health conditions such as diabetes, congestive heart failure (CHF), chronic obstructive pulmonary disease (COPD), or Crohn's disease, the Navigator's influence becomes even more significant. Again, acting as both advocate and educator, the Navigator develops a deep understanding of the nuances of each disease, enabling them to anticipate patient needs and facilitate timely interventions. Their expertise ensures that patients receive proactive support, from monitoring symptoms and coordinating specialist appointments to educating on medication management and lifestyle adjustments.

By specializing in particular diseases or patient populations, Navigators can identify early warning signs of potential exacerbations and intervene before these issues escalate into acute crises. This sustained involvement promotes adherence to treatment regimens and empowers patients to take an active role in managing their own health. Throughout these ongoing relationships, Navigators provide ongoing encouragement and clear guidance, helping patients navigate complex healthcare systems, access community resources, and maintain continuity of care.

The Navigator's comprehensive approach supports patients in following the trajectory of their illness, minimizing hospitalizations, and improving overall quality of life while fostering a sense of confidence and self-efficacy in patients and their families.

A key part of the Navigator role is to stay abreast of current leading practices as it relates to both the surgical and medical conditions of patients as well as any changes in regulations to align the care and education for both the provider offices and the patients.

3.6 Special Populations and Specific Needs

One of the most rewarding and challenging aspects of Case Management is working with diverse populations, each with their unique set of challenges. Case Managers must be culturally competent and equipped to handle the specific needs of various demographics. This may include working with elderly patients, individuals with developmental disabilities, or those with chronic illnesses. Each group may have distinct barriers to care due to socioeconomic factors, literacy levels, cultural beliefs, or accessibility issues.

For instance, managing care for elderly patients may involve coordinating transportation services for medical appointments, while for younger adults, it might mean connecting them with vocational training programs to promote independence. Understanding Social Drivers of Health (SDOH) and Health-Related Health Needs (HRHN), like income, education, and access to resources, is vital for Case Managers to address factors that impact patient health outcomes. Adopting a holistic approach allows Case Managers to support patients beyond clinical needs, considering the entire spectrum of their lived experiences.

3.7 Education and Training for Future Generations

In addition to their coordination responsibilities, Case Managers also assume the role of educators. As the specialty of Case Management continues to evolve, there is a growing need for experts in the field to educate and train the next generation of Case Managers. This educational component is not only beneficial for patients and their families but also contributes to the overall growth and advancement of the healthcare industry.

Experts emphasize the importance of formal training and mentorship pathways for new Case Managers. Comprehensive training programs that cover essential skills, including communication, time management, and conflict resolution, can profoundly impact the effectiveness of Case Management. Hospitals and organizations should consider investing in ongoing professional development and continuing education opportunities, which can improve job satisfaction for Case Managers and enhance patient care quality.

3.8 The Evolving Future of Case Management

Looking ahead, the future of Case Management is both exciting and promising. As healthcare needs diversify, new roles and settings will continue to emerge, ensuring that patients receive the highest quality of care while adapting to changing environments. Innovative models of care, like integrated care teams and Patient-Centered Medical Homes (PCMH), emphasize the importance of comprehensive Case Management.

As the healthcare landscape continues to shift, it is evident that the roles of Utilization Review and Case Managers will become increasingly scrutinized by executive leadership teams, particularly concerning patient throughput management. An organization's financial health often relies on efficient use of resources and technology-backed case management practices. Understanding the foundational aspects of each role and the standard practices associated with them will enhance the efficiency and effectiveness of healthcare teams.

3.9 Adapting to Change

In the face of regulatory changes, technological advancements, and the ever-evolving needs of patients, Case Managers must exhibit flexibility and readiness to adapt. This adaptability will be a key component in ensuring that healthcare systems remain patient-centered and effective while also being cost-efficient. Implementing best practices, leveraging technology, and continuously seeking out education will ensure Case Managers can rise to the challenges presented by the changing healthcare landscape.

The pivotal role of Case Managers within the healthcare continuum cannot be overstated. They are integral not only in navigating complex systems that patients face but also in driving improvements to the care delivery model as a whole. By enhancing communication, fostering collaboration, and embracing technology, they play a vital role in shaping positive patient outcomes while improving the overall health of communities. As healthcare continues to evolve, the skills and expertise of Case Managers will be essential in ensuring that each patient's journey is one of strength, support, and success. Ultimately, the promise of integrated, patient-centered care rests on the shoulders of these dedicated professionals committed to making a difference in the lives of those they serve.

The following sections will delve deeper into these roles, providing valuable tools and insights to support the functionality and effectiveness of Case Management throughout the healthcare continuum.

3.10 Case Study

Coordination Across the Healthcare Continuum

A 43-year-old patient is being discharged from the hospital post-treatment for a closed head injury. The patient is being transferred to an Inpatient Rehabilitation Hospital for continued care. As part of the discharge process, the Case Manager completes the Transition of Care document, which is sent to the Primary Care Provider's office.

After completing the inpatient rehab stay, the patient is referred to for ongoing outpatient therapy. The rehabilitation Case Manager assists with the referral process, provides the information to the outpatient provider selected by the patient, and completes the Transfer of Care document to share with the Primary Care Provider (PCP).

The patient has regular scheduled follow-up appointments with their PCP. The office Care Coordinator assisted the patient in arranging community services for transportation due to the limitation placed on driving.

Upon the 6-month visit, the patient is diagnosed with a condition that is unrelated to the head injury, requiring a return to the hospital. Upon arranging for the patient's transportation to the hospital, the office Care Coordinator contacted the hospital's Case Management department to provide information regarding office care, community services arranged, and the current home health agency providing in-house assistance.

Does this communication potentially impact patient care?

This communication will have a positive impact on the care provided for the patient. Clear communication between all healthcare providers seeing a patient reduces the opportunity for care misalignment.

Roles of the Utilization Review Team

4

Learning Objectives

1. **Understanding Utilization Review**: Identify the key responsibilities and functions of the Utilization Review (UR) team within the healthcare system.
2. **Importance in Revenue Cycle:** Recognize the critical role of UR in the Revenue Integrity Cycle and its impact on financial health for healthcare organizations.
3. **Clinical Documentation:** Learn the significance of accurate and effective clinical documentation and communication between payors and providers to ensure appropriate payment for services.
4. **Understanding Denial Management:** Explain the importance of a well-organized denial management strategy and identify key components that contribute to its effectiveness.
5. **Continuous Education:** Emphasize the importance of staying updated on national criteria guidelines, payor requirements, and regulatory changes to maintain compliance and best practices within the UR function.
6. **Interdisciplinary Collaboration:** Highlight the collaborative role that the UR team plays in fostering communication among healthcare providers, payors, and other stakeholders to enhance patient care outcomes.
7. **Payor Relations:** Discuss the significance of building strong relationships between the Utilization Review (UR) team and payor organizations, highlighting the benefits of ongoing engagement and communication.

In recent years, healthcare leaders have increasingly acknowledged the critical role of Utilization Review (UR) staff within the broader healthcare system. Recognizing their importance has led to enhanced support for their functioning and staffing, along

S. Garceau, *Interdisciplinary Case Management: A Nursing Practice Approach*,
https://doi.org/10.1007/978-3-032-20960-3_4

with the implementation of process improvement initiatives. As a result, the UR team has become an indispensable part of the Revenue Integrity Cycle, working diligently to ensure that healthcare delivery is both efficient and effective.

The UR team plays a significant role in initiating clinical conversations with payors, helping to secure payment for services rendered to patients. Their responsibilities extend beyond merely ensuring payment; they are accountable to guarantee that accurate and relevant clinical information is documented and effectively communicated with both payors and providers. This communication is vital for improving the quality of care delivered to each patient. To uphold a high level of professionalism and to ensure compliance with industry standards, UR staff must stay abreast of the latest national criteria guidelines, payor requirements, and regulations set forth by the Centers for Medicare & Medicaid Services (CMS). Keeping up with these changes is not just beneficial but essential for maintaining best practices and compliance within the healthcare environment.

The role of UR staff is particularly crucial in the context of denial management, a pressing concern in modern healthcare. Denials can have significant financial ramifications for healthcare providers, leading to delayed payments and increased administrative burdens. As the first line of defense in denial mitigation efforts, UR staff play a pivotal role in the Revenue Integrity Cycle. By proactively engaging in the review process while a patient is still under the care of a provider, the UR team can significantly influence the clarity of the information shared with payors. This proactive approach not only facilitates timely communication between the payor and the patient's provider or designated representative, but it also ensures that potential issues are addressed before they escalate into more significant problems.

To optimize their effectiveness, it is crucial to establish a streamlined work process that enables the Utilization Review team to manage their caseloads efficiently. An effective workflow allows staff to prioritize tasks, structure their day effectively, and avoid duplicating efforts or missing critical steps in the patient record processing. To achieve this, it's essential for the team to review the daily schedule or census and identify the following categories of cases: new cases, cases that require follow-up in accordance with policy or payor requests, and cases necessitating authorization of services from payors.

A best practice for the UR team begins with prioritizing new cases that have not yet undergone review. This practice aids in managing patient throughput effectively while ensuring sound financial management for business operations, including timely communication with payors. In this context, observation cases should be processed first, followed by inpatient admissions, to align with both clinical needs and operational efficiency.

Additionally, it is essential for the UR team to utilize effective documentation techniques to ensure that all communications and actions are accurately recorded. Maintaining a comprehensive record not only supports compliance but also enhances the ability to appeal denials successfully should they occur. Documentation serves as a means to capture the reasoning behind clinical decisions and payor interactions, which is vital in the event of future audits or disputes.

To maintain compliance with CMS standards and the specific requirements of various payors, implementing a standardized process that delineates the frequency of reviews is vital. Each payor may have different contractual agreements regarding concurrent reviews. Thus, integrating these requirements into the UR team's concurrent or continued stay review policy is essential. This adherence not only ensures continued authorization for patient admissions but also plays a significant role in mitigating potential denials.

The next step towards a more effective and efficient utilization review process involves thoroughly reviewing cases that require outstanding payor authorizations. Engaging in open communication with the payor's UR team is necessary to obtain the required authorizations and actively work towards mitigating any potential denials before they occur. Collaborating effectively with payors can create a more transparent relationship, reducing misunderstandings, and fostering a more efficient authorization process.

Implementing a structured approach ensures that all cases receive appropriate coverage from the UR team without overburdening staff. This not only eases workflow but also guarantees that accurate reviews and processes are consistently followed. Including ongoing training and education for UR staff is critical. Regularly scheduled training sessions can help the team stay current with changes in healthcare regulations, payor policies, and best practices, ensuring that they remain effective in their roles.

In the subsequent sections, detailed workflow processes will be provided as a foundational framework that can be tailored to meet the specific needs of individual providers and their teams. These processes, which have been refined and updated over many years, will serve as templates that can be adapted as necessary. Given the ever-evolving healthcare landscape, the commitment to continuous improvement and adaptation will remain imperative. By establishing robust processes, healthcare organizations can ensure that the right steps are taken at the right time and that the appropriate resources are utilized efficiently to optimize both patient care and financial outcomes.

By focusing on quality, compliance, and efficiency, the UR team can significantly contribute to the overall success of healthcare organizations. This not only enhances the financial health of the organization but ultimately leads to better patient outcomes. Improving the utilization review process is an ongoing journey that requires teamwork, communication, and a steadfast dedication to excellence in healthcare.

4.1 Point of Entry Utilization Management

The integration of Utilization Review (UR) into every point of entry for patients within the healthcare system is pivotal for ensuring timely and effective evaluation of care needs. Utilization Review serves as a systematic process designed to assess the necessity, appropriateness, and efficiency of the healthcare services provided to patients. By embedding UR processes at critical junctures—such as during scheduled surgical and procedural services, direct admissions from community or provider offices, and transfers from external facilities or emergency departments—we can significantly enhance the quality and efficiency of care offered to patients.

When UR is incorporated at these critical touchpoints, healthcare providers can manage resources more effectively. This approach not only helps in minimizing unnecessary costs but also ensures that patients receive the most appropriate care in a timely manner, thus improving overall health outcomes. Additionally, implementing UR at the entry points allows for proactive identification of patients who may require more intensive resources or specialized services, ultimately leading to a more streamlined care delivery process. Coupled with efficient communication between various healthcare teams, this creates a holistic framework aimed at optimizing patient care and resource allocation across the healthcare spectrum.

Point of Entry: Surgical and Procedural Areas

Integrating Utilization Review (UR) into surgical and procedural areas plays a crucial role in enhancing the quality of patient care while simultaneously optimizing operational efficiency within healthcare settings. This integration not only focuses on confirming the medical necessity of procedures but also supports the determination of the appropriate level of care required for each patient. It ensures that patients receive the most suitable treatment environment tailored to their specific medical needs.

Every patient presents unique medical histories, individual needs, and varying risk factors that must be considered carefully. By implementing UR practices, healthcare providers can thoroughly assess these elements, which helps ensure that decisions regarding patient placement in surgical or procedural settings are grounded in a comprehensive understanding of their condition. This careful evaluation process ultimately aims to maximize the potential for successful outcomes, thereby providing patients with the best possible chance for recovery and overall health improvement.

The integration of UR aligns with the operational goals of hospitals and surgical centers. By effectively identifying patients who may benefit from alternative care settings, whether that be outpatient services, outpatient surgery centers, or other less intensive environments, healthcare facilities can streamline their resources. This not only helps manage costs but also allows for a greater focus on patients who truly require higher levels of intervention. Such a targeted approach enhances the overall efficacy of care delivery.

The systematic use of UR can lead to improved patient satisfaction, as it ensures that care is more personalized and responsive to each individual's needs. Patients who feel that their specific situations are understood and addressed are often more engaged in their treatment plans. Implementing a thoughtful and systematic application of Utilization Review within surgical and procedural areas is integral to fostering an environment where patient care is prioritized through individualized assessment and evidence-based decision-making.

This dedicated approach not only bolsters the quality of care provided but also supports the sustainable operational health of healthcare institutions, ultimately benefiting patients, providers, and the broader medical community alike. Ultimately, a well-executed UR process contributes significantly to the advancement of healthcare standards, ensuring that the focus remains on achieving the best outcomes for all involved (Fig. 4.1).

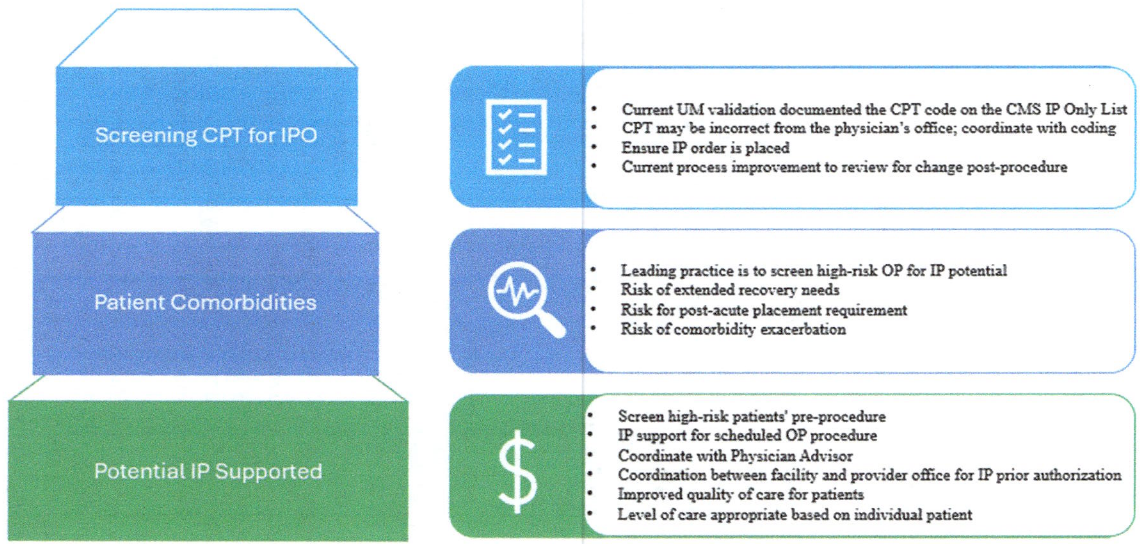

Fig. 4.1 Highlights of key areas included in documentation to review as part of procedural utilization review. Created by the author

Point of Entry: Transfer

When a patient is transferred from one level of care, such as a long-term care facility to an acute care hospital, it is essential to thoroughly assess the medical necessity for admission. This process involves a detailed review of the patient's medical history and current condition, ensuring that the receiving facility can provide the appropriate and required level of care needed for the patient's specific situation.

Effective communication with the transferring providers is crucial in obtaining necessary documentation and insights into the patient's treatment needs. This communication not only helps with the continuity of care but also ensures that all parties involved are aware of the patient's medical details and any urgent concerns that may require immediate attention. Additionally, the objective review of the documentation supporting the patient's medical necessity is critical. This includes evaluating plans for repatriation at the conclusion of specialized services and determining the medical appropriateness for discharge back to services in the patient's home area.

The role of the Utilization Review (UR) nurse is significant in this process. UR nurses assist in facilitating the transfer by ensuring that all documentation is in order and initiating effective communication with the payor source as well as the multidisciplinary care team. This coordination is essential for smooth transition planning and for making sure that the patient continues to receive high-quality care as they move between different levels of care. By overseeing this transition, UR nurses play a pivotal role in ensuring the patient's health outcomes are optimized and that all healthcare services are appropriately utilized.

Point of Entry: Direct Admission

Direct admissions play a crucial role in healthcare management by allowing patients to be admitted directly to a hospital or facility from outpatient clinics or physicians' offices, thereby bypassing the often lengthy and resource-intensive process of an Emergency Department visit. This innovative approach not only enhances the overall patient experience but also optimizes hospital resources, ultimately improving overall efficiency in patient care delivery.

When a direct admission occurs, one of the key steps is to ensure that all relevant documentation is promptly obtained. This includes comprehensive medical records, test results, and any notes from the attending physician that detail the patient's condition and the necessity for hospitalization. These documents are vital for a thorough review of medical necessity, which helps in determining whether the level of care being provided aligns with what is clinically justified. The accuracy and completeness of documentation can significantly influence patient outcomes, as they ensure the medical team has all necessary information to make informed decisions.

Communication with the attending provider is equally essential to accurately convey the patient's status to the payor source. This alignment ensures that the reason for admission and the anticipated level of care are clearly understood by all parties involved, facilitating a smoother authorization process for reimbursement. Securing this authorization is critical, as it directly impacts the financial viability of the hospital and the ability to provide ongoing care for patients. Without proper authorization, both the institution and the patient may face significant financial burdens, highlighting the importance of thorough preparation during the admission process.

Implementing effective direct admission protocols can lead to several substantial benefits. By reducing the need for Emergency Department visits, healthcare facilities can streamline patient flow, leading to shorter wait times and enhanced patient satisfaction. This efficient process also fosters better continuity of care, as patients can be seen and managed by their healthcare providers in a more structured and timely manner. Additionally, when handled effectively, direct admissions can result in significant cost savings for both healthcare facilities and patients by minimizing unnecessary diagnostic tests and procedures typically associated with emergency visits.

Direct admissions, when executed properly, create a win-win scenario for patients and healthcare providers alike. They not only improve the overall quality of care but also enhance the operational efficiency of healthcare institutions, leading to better health outcomes and reduced expenses. By prioritizing direct admissions as a strategy for patient management, healthcare systems can effectively navigate the complexities of patient care while promoting a more positive experience for everyone involved.

Point of Entry: Admission via the Emergency Department or Free-standing Emergency Centers

Admissions through the Emergency Department (ED) or free-standing emergency centers necessitate a thorough evaluation of medical necessity due to the often unpredictable nature of ED visits. These environments are characterized by high acuity and varied patient presentations, which can complicate the admission process. Utilization Review (UR) staff within the ED play a critical role and should focus intently on the screening documentation that identifies the severity of the patient's condition and supports the rationale for admission. This evaluation process requires effective collaboration with the attending provider and, when needed, the physician advisor. This teamwork ensures that the level of care is properly determined based on the physician's clinical judgment, which reflects the patient's condition and circumstances as documented in the medical record.

The complexities inherent in the ED environment necessitate that UR staff possess a comprehensive understanding of various medical conditions and the nuances of emergency care protocols. They must be adept at rapidly assessing patient needs and making informed decisions that align with both clinical best practices and payor requirements. Each insurance provider has its own set of requirements and policies regarding admissions from ED settings. This adds another layer of complexity that UR nurses must navigate. They need to be well-versed in these specific guidelines to effectively communicate with payors and justify an admission based on the established criteria. Their expertise is important not just for ensuring that admissions are necessary and appropriate, but also for facilitating a smooth transition from the emergency setting to inpatient care when warranted.

The UR staff must stay current with evolving healthcare regulations and policies, which can impact admission criteria and documentation standards. Regular training and professional development are essential to maintain proficiency in these areas. By staying informed and adaptable, UR staff can provide the best possible support to patients and healthcare providers, ensuring seamless and efficient admissions processes that promote optimal patient outcomes.

The role of UR staff in the ED is multifaceted and requires a comprehensive understanding of clinical practices, insurance requirements, and the dynamics of emergency medicine to ensure the best outcomes for patients while also satisfying administrative and financial considerations.

Working collaboratively with admitting providers, UR will ensure that patients are placed in the most appropriate level of care and followed for appropriate throughput management. Communicating this information promptly with payors will also support reimbursement more judiciously.

In free-standing emergency centers, the role of UR staff is equally critical. These centers often serve as the first point of contact for patients requiring immediate medical attention. UR staff must be proficient in handling admissions, coordinating with various departments, and managing patient transfers when higher levels of care are needed. Their expertise in insurance verification, authorization processes, and documentation standards is invaluable in preventing delays and facilitating smooth transitions.

4.2 Important Role for Utilization Review Integration

Integration of Utilization Review (UR) processes is crucial across all portals of entry. Education for staff on UR principles and how they align with national guidelines can enhance understanding of what constitutes medical necessity. The UR staff must be familiar with the documentation review processes and adherence to the Conditions of Participation and scope of licensure concerns. Open communication with physicians, other providers, and engagement of the Physician Advisor are crucial to the point of entry UR process. Staff also needs a deep understanding of the potential financial ramifications for both patients and facilities if admissions do not meet UR criteria as well as physician clinical determination, thereby highlighting the impact on patient satisfaction and care quality.

UR staff play a pivotal role in patient advocacy, ensuring that individuals receive the necessary care without undue financial burdens. They must stay informed about changes in insurance policies, coverage options, and healthcare regulations to provide accurate guidance and support to patients and their families.

A proactive approach to Utilization Review can amplify patient outcomes. By identifying care needs early, health providers can implement preventive measures and initiate timely interventions, ultimately leading to a more favorable recovery trajectory for patients. Additionally, by focusing on appropriate levels of care, UR promotes a more efficient healthcare delivery model that not only reduces costs but also alleviates pressure on healthcare systems.

Also, regular assessments and monitoring through Utilization Review ensure that patients receive the most appropriate treatments tailored to their individual needs. This personalized care approach can significantly enhance patient satisfaction and improve overall health outcomes. By optimizing resource allocation and minimizing unnecessary procedures, UR also contributes to the sustainability of the healthcare system. Effective communication among healthcare teams, facilitated by Utilization Review, ensures that care plans are consistently updated and adapted to the evolving needs of patients, fostering a collaborative environment that ultimately benefits patient care.

4.3 Financial Impact on Patients and Facilities

Understanding the financial implications of admissions is essential for all staff. Educational programs should address how medical necessity influences reimbursement rates for facilities and out-of-pocket costs for patients. Staff should be trained to communicate effectively with patients about their insurance options and what they can expect regarding coverage and billing. This knowledge empowers healthcare providers to advocate for patients and navigate the complexities of healthcare financing, ultimately improving overall patient experience and satisfaction.

By expanding on these areas, we can ensure that healthcare providers are well-equipped to manage patient admissions effectively, advocate for patients' financial well-being, and maintain compliance with insurance requirements.

4.4 Observation Management

Observation management is a critical aspect of patient care that requires thoughtful consideration and a keen understanding of various care levels. This often misunderstood status can be prone to either overuse or underuse in many healthcare facilities, highlighting the need for a more structured approach. Best practices dictate that the right patient is placed in the appropriate observation status at the right time during their hospital stay. This necessitates ongoing scrutiny and assessment of observation status cases, ideally conducted at least twice daily. Such regular reviews help determine whether conditions warrant an upgrade to inpatient status based on comprehensive documentation and clinical criteria (Fig. 4.2).

A key aspect of effective observation management involves the collaboration between Utilization Review (UR) teams and the Physician Advisor (PA) or UR provider. Conducting rapid observation rounds twice daily facilitates timely management of cases and allows for quick escalation when necessary. These huddles play an essential role in confirming that patients are being closely monitored and that their care is adjusted as needed.

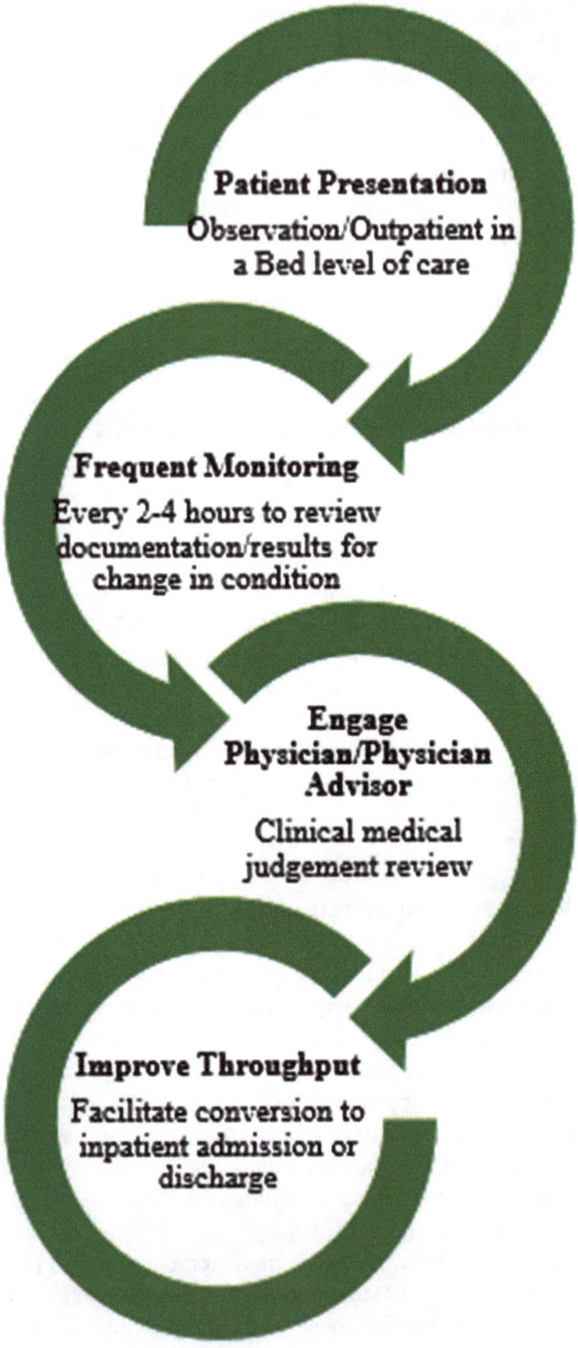

Fig. 4.2 Observation management requires a methodical approach to reviewing records for this population of patients. Created by the author

During observation rounds, healthcare providers engage in a thorough review of each patient's progress, assess any fluctuations in their condition, and identify potential barriers to a timely discharge. This collaborative approach not only ensures that the patients receive the appropriate level of care but also allows for any necessary adjustments to be implemented swiftly. By regularly reassessing patients' needs and statuses, healthcare teams can reduce the risks associated with unmet healthcare requirements.

Active observation management provides a safeguard against unnecessary hospital admissions, which can be both costly and resource-draining. It promotes efficient resource utilization by distinguishing between patients who require intensive inpatient care and those who can be managed with a less restrictive observation status. This differentiation is crucial for optimizing patient flow and ensuring hospital resources are allocated appropriately. By fostering a culture of continuous assessment and collaborative decision-making, healthcare facilities can enhance patient outcomes and ensure that each patient receives care tailored to their specific needs at every stage of their hospital journey.

4.5 Expanding on Focused Observation Rounds

Focused observation rounds present a significant opportunity to enhance communication between healthcare providers, patients, and their families. Care teams can leverage these interactions by engaging patients in meaningful discussions about their care plans, answering any questions, and addressing a variety of concerns. This approach fosters a supportive environment that is conducive to healing and satisfaction. When patients and their families are actively involved in these conversations, they tend to feel more empowered and informed about their healthcare journey. Research shows that when patients understand their treatment options and the rationale behind care decisions, their overall satisfaction increases. This enhancement of patient satisfaction is not merely a matter of comfort; it often translates into improved health outcomes as well. Informed and engaged patients are better equipped to follow treatment protocols, adhere to medication regimens, and actively participate in their recovery, which ultimately contributes to better health outcomes.

The focused observation rounds also serve an educational purpose for healthcare teams. These rounds reinforce the critical importance of adhering to best practices in clinical guidelines and documentation standards. As team members share their insights and experiences during these rounds, they have the chance to learn from one another, gaining awareness of various approaches to patient care. This continuous sharing of knowledge and critical reflection fosters an atmosphere of growth and improvement, which is essential for any healthcare setting aiming to provide high-quality care.

Time and again, studies indicate that collaboration among healthcare professionals—such as physicians, nurses, case managers, and social workers—can substantially elevate the quality of care provided. By engaging in focused observation rounds, healthcare teams create a structured forum to discuss not just patient care challenges, but also potential solutions. These discussions can lead to the implementation of new strategies designed to enhance patient outcomes and streamline care delivery processes.

4.6 Implementing Rapid Observation Rounds

The implementation of rapid observation rounds is crucial for effective observation management. This structured approach allows healthcare providers to assess patient conditions quickly and efficiently while maintaining a focus on collaboration. By gathering interdisciplinary teams—comprising various healthcare professionals—and encouraging open dialogue with patients and their families, the rapid observation rounds can significantly influence the trajectory of care.

In particular, having a dedicated Utilization Review (UR) facilitator can help streamline these rounds. The UR facilitator plays a pivotal role by maintaining a focus on ensuring that all care provided is medically necessary, and that it aligns with both clinical guidelines and hospital policies. Facilitation of communication between the clinical staff, patients, and families helps create a more cohesive healthcare experience. The synergy developed during these rounds allows for timely interventions that can prevent complications and reduce length of stay.

A crucial part of this process occurs during the morning and afternoon observation rounds. Morning rounds typically involve a comprehensive review of patient cases, allowing the team to prepare for the day ahead. These rounds include attending discussions about inpatient orders requested, pending tests, utilization review monitoring, and any potential discharge needs that might have arisen. In the afternoon, another dedicated meeting allows team members to evaluate the results from the morning rounds, assess new cases, and address any urgent needs for testing, treatments, or discharge planning.

In this way, observation rounds serve as an integral tool for communication, education, and the overall enhancement of inpatient care.

4.7 Strengthening Inpatient Utilization Management

Inpatient management represents a cornerstone of contemporary healthcare delivery, requiring an intricate tapestry of collaboration among various teams to ensure that patient care is both efficient and effective. Among the most significant collaborations is the synergy between the Utilization Review (UR) team and the Clinical Documentation Integrity (CDI) team. This partnership is vital, as it directly aligns medical necessity with the appropriate diagnostic-related group (DRG) assignment.

The UR team plays a critical role in evaluating whether the care provided to patients is necessary during their hospital stay. To achieve this, they must ensure that all the services rendered meet established criteria for medical necessity. This evaluation must closely synchronize with the CDI team, which focuses on ensuring that clinical documentation accurately reflects patients' diagnoses and the complexities of their conditions. The relationship between these teams is essential for guaranteeing compliant documentation that adheres to coding requirements, which in turn impacts hospital reimbursement rates and resource allocation.

Accurate documentation directly influences DRG assignment categorization used to determine payment for hospital cases. The DRG system is paramount for sustaining hospital operations; an accurate DRG assignment facilitates appropriate reimbursement and resources, enabling hospitals to maintain financial viability while providing quality care to patients.

Coordination between the UR and CDI teams permits healthcare providers to accurately assess the geometric length of stay (GLOS) or geometric mean length of stay (GMLOS) for each patient. Communicating this information effectively to both the care team and unit case managers is crucial for managing the progression of each patient's care. Understanding the GLOS/GMLOS helps the care team predict how long patients should ideally remain hospitalized based on their diagnoses and treatment plans. Armed with this information, the team can more effectively manage patient care, streamline treatment protocols, anticipate discharge planning needs, and allocate resources accordingly.

4.8 Coordinating with Other Teams

Within healthcare, often departments become focused on their specific roles, responsibilities, accountabilities and reporting. However, with the current healthcare environment, it is becoming more important to work in a collaborative relationship with all other departments within the facility.

Case Management, Utilization Management, and Clinical Documentation Integrity fill a very unique role as they are all included in the clinical care team as well as the revenue cycle and business team. Transparency and sharing valuable information between the two teams is key for these teams.

Aligning the three departments with open communication pathways is the first step on this journey.

4.9 The Role of Collaboration in Clinical Documentation Integrity (CDI)

A collaborative approach fosters a holistic perspective on inpatient management, ensuring that every aspect of a patient's care is considered and accounted for. This integration facilitates improved clinical outcomes, as healthcare professionals can more rapidly identify potential hurdles in a patient's recovery. When challenges arise, rapid team coordination can lead to the timely implementation of strategies that ensure effective and efficient discharge when appropriate.

The partnership between Utilization Review and Clinical Documentation Integrity teams is not merely a procedural necessity; it is integral to optimizing inpatient management. This collaboration engenders a shared commitment to compliance with medical necessity requirements while also enhancing the overall quality of care provided to patients during their stay. Ensuring that documentation accurately reflects both the patient's condition and the services rendered is crucial when advocating for patients' rights to receive appropriate healthcare.

4.10 Strategic Coordination with the Care Team

The role of Utilization Review in patient throughput and care management within hospital settings cannot be overstated, even if it is often overlooked. The information generated through the UR process has a directly substantial impact on the efficiency of patient flow throughout the hospital system. Each patient's care status determines how quickly and effectively they can transition through various stages of their hospital journey.

Understanding each patient's level of care status is essential for effective discharge planning and coordinated care. By meticulously assessing patients' individual needs and meticulously documenting their cases, healthcare professionals can facilitate timely discharges that align with organizational length of stay management goals. For example, observation cases often necessitate a discharge within 48 h of admission to optimize resource utilization. In contrast, inpatient stays may require longer recovery periods based on the complexities of the patient's clinical condition.

A well-structured approach to patient management through utilization review provides a roadmap for transitioning patients systematically through various phases of care. Coordinated communication helps to ensure that care is not only delivered effectively but is also documented properly, creating an environment where healthcare providers can focus on delivering the best possible outcomes for their patients.

4.11 Enhancing Team Collaboration

In practice, this might involve regular interdisciplinary meetings wherein UR professionals, case managers, nurses, and physicians gather to review active cases, discuss ongoing patient needs, and coordinate future care plans. Utilizing a structured agenda for these meetings can help keep discussions focused and ensure that all relevant topics are covered, leading to clearer communication and more effective decision-making.

Through this collaborative process, each team member can bring their unique perspectives and expertise to the table, allowing for more comprehensive patient assessments and collectively developed care strategies. Engaging in open dialogue fosters an atmosphere of trust and cooperation, which is indispensable for instilling a culture of excellence within the healthcare environment.

As patients and their families are increasingly participating in their own care, their insights and experiences can be an invaluable addition to these meetings. Soliciting patient and family feedback encourages a patient-centered approach to care, ultimately leading to higher levels of satisfaction and better clinical outcomes.

4.12 Continuous Improvement and Adaptation

The need for continuous improvement cannot be overstated in a rapidly evolving healthcare landscape. A proactive approach is essential for addressing the dynamic nature of patient care and the complexity of the healthcare environment. This entails regularly revisiting and refining existing protocols, processes, and communication strategies to enhance the overall quality of care provided.

Healthcare organizations should engage in regular training sessions to reinforce the importance of compliance with utilization review guidelines and ensure that all team members are familiar with updated practices and policies. Continuous education can also include sharing case studies and discussing different strategies employed in handling various patient scenarios. Encouraging professional development through ongoing learning opportunities helps cultivate experts within the team who can contribute effectively to patient care and operational efficiency.

By fostering an environment that values improvement, dialogue, and education, organizations can position themselves to respond more effectively to changes in patient needs and systemic challenges. Such a focus on improvement not only leads to better patient care but also enables healthcare systems to thrive amidst the shifting challenges of the industry.

4.13 Denial Management

To achieve this synergy, it's imperative to establish open lines of communication and regular meetings among these key players. By sharing insights and discussing case studies, the UR team, CM, and CDI specialists can collectively identify patterns and potential areas for improvement. This unified approach ensures that when a case is reviewed, all aspects of the patient's condition are thoroughly documented, and the medical necessity is clearly articulated.

The processes outlined previously demonstrate that concurrent denial mitigation efforts are intricately woven into the workflows. This integration is particularly significant for the Utilization Review team, as it enhances the likelihood of successfully overturning denials. Engaging physicians and Physician Advisors (PA) during this ongoing care process allows for timely documentation improvements, ensuring that the clinical rationale for patient care is clearly articulated and aligned with payor expectations.

Utilization Review serves as the frontline defense in denial management. It is paramount for identifying potential areas where documentation may fall short and highlighting opportunities for process improvements. By proactively addressing these issues, the UR team can significantly reduce the incidence of similar denials in the future. Maintaining thorough documentation of payor-related information tied to denials equips the Revenue Cycle denial management team with critical insights. This data not only aids in recognizing emerging trends but also informs strategic decisions and operational enhancements to facilitate optimal financial outcomes.

Overall, a cohesive approach that integrates UR, CM, and CDI with continued education for clinical staff empowers healthcare organizations to streamline their denial management processes, ultimately improving revenue cycle performance while ensuring high-quality patient care.

4.14 Short Stay Review

The Utilization Review (UR) team is tasked with the critical responsibility of evaluating cases that involve admissions with a length of stay of less than 48 h. These short-term admissions are subject to heightened scrutiny from payors, as they raise questions about the necessity and appropriateness of inpatient care provided. It's essential for the UR team to conduct a thorough examination of each case to validate that the care level rendered was indeed warranted, relying heavily on comprehensive documentation and adherence to established exclusionary criteria.

Exclusionary criteria are specific circumstances that necessitate inpatient-level care, regardless of how brief the stay may be. The UR team should be well-versed in these criteria to ensure accurate assessments. Some notable examples include:

CMS Inpatient-Only Procedures: Certain medical procedures are designated by the Centers for Medicare & Medicaid Services (CMS) as requiring inpatient hospitalization. Any patient undergoing such procedures qualifies for inpatient status, regardless of the duration of their hospital stay.

Patient Transfers for Specialized Care to Another Acute Care Setting: Admissions that involve transferring a patient to another acute care hospital for specialized interventions, treatment, or surgery must be recognized as clinically justified, thus qualifying for inpatient care.

Patient Expiration: In the unfortunate event of a patient's death during their hospital stay, the admission is deemed necessary and should be classified as meeting the criteria for inpatient-level care.

Leave Against Medical Advice (AMA): If a patient decides to leave the hospital against medical advice, the UR team must examine the details surrounding this decision to determine if inpatient care was justified prior to their departure.

Transition to Hospice or Comfort Measures: Situations where a patient's condition necessitates a shift to hospice care or palliative measures clearly warrant a higher level of care, regardless of the duration of the stay.

Rapid Patient Recovery: Documented evidence showing that a patient has recovered more quickly than anticipated can also serve as an important factor in considering their need for inpatient care.

Initiation of Mechanical Ventilation: Initiation of mechanical ventilation is defined as the commencement of assisted breathing using a mechanical ventilator, typically via an endotracheal tube or other airway device, to support or replace spontaneous respiratory effort. This process is generally indicated when a patient is unable to maintain adequate oxygenation or ventilation on their own due to conditions such as respiratory failure, compromised airway protection, or severe neurological impairment. The clinical documentation should clearly reflect the time and reason for beginning mechanical ventilation, noting all relevant patient assessments and interventions associated with this critical care event.

In conducting these reviews, the UR team must approach each case with diligence, ensuring that all necessary documentation is meticulously evaluated. This not only helps uphold the integrity of patient care but also ensures compliance with payor expectations and regulatory standards. The goal is to facilitate a fair assessment of care that reflects the true needs of the patients while preventing unnecessary denials and enhancing the overall quality of care provided.

Also, it is paramount for the UR team to engage in continuous education and training to stay abreast of evolving guidelines and policies. Regular audits and feedback sessions can help identify areas for improvement in the review process. Collaboration with clinical staff and physicians is also crucial, as their insights and firsthand experiences can provide valuable context to the documentation being reviewed. By fostering a culture of transparency and communication, the UR team can effectively navigate the complexities of short-term admissions and contribute to better patient outcomes.

Additionally, implementing advanced data analytics tools can aid in identifying trends and patterns that may signal potential issues in patient care. These tools can enhance the team's ability to make informed decisions and streamline the review process. Embracing technology not only improves efficiency but also ensures a more comprehensive evaluation of each case.

The UR team's diligent efforts in reviewing short-term admissions are vital in maintaining the integrity of healthcare services. By adhering to exclusionary criteria, engaging in continuous education, collaborating with clinical staff, and leveraging advanced analytics, the UR team can ensure that the level of care provided aligns with the true needs of the patients while meeting regulatory standards and payor expectations.

4.15 Utilization Review is a Key Member of the Revenue Cycle Team

To effectively manage and mitigate denials in healthcare, it is essential to establish a robust and well-defined process that clearly outlines each team member's roles and responsibilities. A well-structured approach involves identifying specific handoff points between teams, which facilitates a seamless transition of tasks and responsibilities, thereby minimizing the risk of errors or delays.

A comprehensive denial management process serves multiple purposes. It not only helps healthcare organizations reduce the frequency of denials but also significantly improves overall revenue cycle performance and enhances patient satisfaction. Given the multifaceted nature of denials, organizations must embrace a proactive and collaborative approach. This entails not only addressing denials as they occur but also implementing preventive measures aimed at reducing their future occurrence.

The collaboration between the Utilization Review team and the Revenue Cycle team is pivotal in managing and mitigating denials effectively. The Utilization Review team performs thorough reviews of all denials, carefully identifying root causes that the facility can address. This proactive analysis allows the organization to implement strategies designed to prevent similar denials in the future. Additionally, the team plays a crucial role in recognizing cases that warrant escalation to contracting departments for negotiation, as well as those denials that fall outside the facility's control and must be managed as they arise. The expertise of the Utilization Review team in evaluating medical necessity and compliance with guidelines is invaluable for ensuring that services provided meet established standards, thereby reducing the likelihood of denials due to non-compliance.

Most denials are indicative of a breakdown or gap in existing processes. To accurately identify where these gaps occur, it is crucial to foster a collaborative team environment. Each team member should be encouraged to analyze the relevant information objectively, engaging in constructive discussions to pinpoint the breakdowns. By working together in this manner, the team can effectively implement targeted improvements that address the identified issues and enhance the denial management process. Continuous education and training for staff members play a vital role in equipping them with the knowledge and skills necessary to navigate complex denial scenarios and apply best practices in their daily operations.

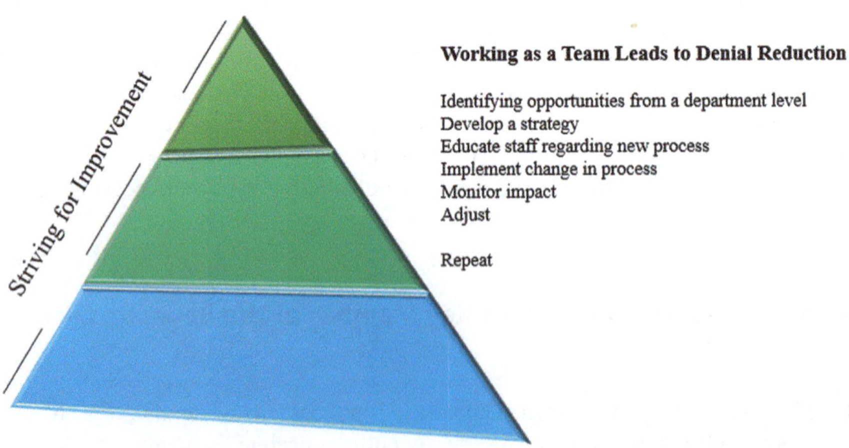

Fig. 4.3 Denial management is not a single process, it is a continuous improvement process. Created by the author

A well-organized denial management strategy that emphasizes clear roles, effective collaboration, and continuous improvement not only reduces denials but also contributes to the overall success of healthcare organizations. By taking a proactive approach and addressing the root causes of denials, organizations can strengthen their revenue cycles and elevate the level of care and satisfaction they provide to patients. Additionally, leveraging technology and data analytics can provide deeper insights into denial patterns and trends, enabling healthcare facilities to make informed decisions and tailor their strategies to address specific issues effectively. A holistic and integrated approach to denial management is essential for optimizing revenue cycle performance and fostering a culture of excellence in patient care (Fig. 4.3).

4.16 Payor Relations

The collaborative relationship between the UR team and payor organizations extends beyond the immediate scope of patient admissions. It involves continuous engagement, regular updates, and strategic discussions aimed at improving care coordination and financial alignment. The UR team stays abreast of evolving policies, regulations, and best practices within the insurance landscape to ensure compliance and optimize patient advocacy efforts.

By leveraging data analytics and patient outcome metrics, the UR team can present compelling evidence to payor organizations, demonstrating the efficacy and necessity of specific treatments and interventions. This data-driven approach not only bolsters the case for coverage but also helps payors understand the long-term benefits of investing in comprehensive patient care.

Additionally, educational initiatives and joint training sessions between the UR team and payor representatives can foster a shared understanding of complex medical conditions and innovative treatment options. These collaborative learning opportunities enhance mutual respect and cooperation, ultimately leading to more informed and patient-centric decision-making processes.

Through these multifaceted engagements, the UR team's dedication to patient advocacy and healthcare excellence is unwavering, ensuring that every patient receives the highest standard of care regardless of the intricacies of their insurance coverage.

4.17 Case Studies

Observation Management

A 51-year-old patient presents to the Emergency Department with a 2-day history of chest pain and increasing shortness of breath accompanied by weakness. The patient has a history of coronary artery disease and hypertension. Vital signs are stable with negative cardiac enzyme lab results. Due to the patient's history and associated symptoms, it is determined that the patient should be admitted to the hospital.

What level of care might be warranted?

Applying national standard criteria, Observation services are appropriate at this time. You will learn more about determining the level of care through criteria-specific education.

During the evening, the patient experiences a significant increase in chest pain, with a repeated EKG performed demonstrating an ST elevation myocardial infarction (STEMI) requiring emergent intervention and transfer to the Intensive Care Unit.

Based on this information, what action would the Utilization Reviewer take?

Contact the attending provider to discuss a conversion to the Inpatient level of care due to the patient's condition. This would be supported by the nationally accepted screening tool which should be applied using the critical care criteria to support the level of services being provided.

Patient Without Medical Necessity Criteria

During Multidisciplinary Rounds, a 66-year-old patient is discussed. The patient is on day 4 of admission for pneumonia. The current condition per the care team is: Therapy states patient is independent with all mobility; Nursing states patient has been off oxygen support for 2 days, tolerating a regular diet; Case Manager shares no needs at present, and patient requesting to be discharged; Provider states that intravenous fluid is to be continued and discharge planned for 2 days.

The Case Manager discusses the case further with the provider after rounds and is informed the patient will require an additional 2 days. The Case Manager ensures that the Utilization Review is completed due to the lack of medical necessity for continued hospital stay and the case is escalated to the Physician Advisor for review.

Why would the case be referred to a Physician Advisor?

Medical necessity may only be determined by a Physician per CMS guidelines. Due to the lack of criteria supporting continued care, the nurse will engage a secondary physician for review and a peer-to-peer conversation if warranted.

Denial Appeal

The Utilization Review nurse is informed of a denial from a payor for a current hospital patient.

What steps should the Utilization Review nurse take?

The nurse should review all documentation of the completed review, complete a new review, if necessary, then contact the payor UR nurse to discuss the case, offering additional clinical information for review to complete a reconsideration appeal step. If that is unsuccessful, discuss with the attending provider or the Physician Advisor to attempt a peer-to-peer appeal with the Medical Director.

Once a written denial has been received, the hospital has the opportunity for a formal written appeal.

5 Roles Within Case Management to Support Patient Throughput

Learning Objectives

1. **Understanding the Role of Case Management:** Recognize the importance of Case Management in healthcare and how it integrates the skills of both nurses and social workers to enhance patient care.
2. **Collaborative Team Approach:** Identify the benefits of a multidisciplinary approach in Case Management, including effective communication and teamwork among healthcare professionals.
3. **Patient Care Coordination:** Learn how Case Managers facilitate timely and appropriate care by coordinating medical services and monitoring patient outcomes throughout the healthcare journey.
4. **Patient Advocacy:** Describe the role of the CM team in advocating for patients, navigating complex medical conditions, and providing patient education and services to ensure optimal care.
5. **Emotional and Psychological Support:** Explore the role of Case Managers in providing emotional and psychological support to patients, helping them navigate their healthcare experiences.
6. **Collaboration with Other Healthcare Professionals:** Learn about the importance of engaging with physicians, nurses, therapists, and other professionals to create a cohesive care plan that benefits patients.
7. **Interdisciplinary Collaboration in Case Management:** Compare and contrast the roles of nurses and social workers within case management, emphasizing how their collaboration supports overall patient throughput and care coordination.

S. Garceau, *Interdisciplinary Case Management: A Nursing Practice Approach*,
https://doi.org/10.1007/978-3-032-20960-3_5

Case Management is a vital healthcare specialty that integrates the diverse skills and knowledge of both nurses and social workers. This collaborative team approach enhances the overall patient experience and improves healthcare outcomes. Initially centered around discharge planning, the scope of Case Management has significantly broadened to encompass a variety of essential functions that contribute to comprehensive healthcare management.

The primary function of Case Management teams is to ensure that patients receive timely and appropriate care throughout their healthcare journey. This encompasses a wide range of responsibilities, including the coordination of medical services, monitoring patient outcomes, and providing emotional and psychological support to patients and their families. Additionally, Case Managers play a crucial role in developing individualized care plans that align with patients' specific needs and preferences. The collaborative nature of their work necessitates close engagement with physicians, nurses, therapists, and other healthcare professionals, fostering a multidisciplinary approach to patient care.

Nurse case managers and social workers both play crucial roles in the healthcare system, particularly in case management, but their responsibilities and areas of expertise differ significantly.

Similar to the Utilization Review (UR) team, which establishes efficient work processes that prevent team overload, the Case Management team must also implement strategies that optimize their workflow. By structuring their day effectively, they can prioritize essential tasks and minimize duplication of effort while ensuring that no critical steps in patient management are overlooked.

To begin their daily operations, Case Managers should conduct a thorough review of the day's schedule or census. This involves identifying new cases, patients scheduled for discharge that day, and those anticipated for discharge the following day. By doing so, Case Managers can effectively prioritize their workload, ensuring that all patients receive thorough screenings and assessments in compliance with the Conditions of Participation.

After completing the initial review and addressing the most pressing cases, Case Managers become available to assist patients, families, and staff who require additional support. They might conduct visits with various patients to facilitate meaningful connections and partnerships, ensuring that those in need feel supported throughout their healthcare experiences.

5.1 Nurse Case Manager Role

Nurse case managers typically have a strong clinical background, which allows them to assess patients' medical needs effectively. They monitor health conditions and coordinate medical treatments, medications, and therapies.

The primary function of the nurse is to ensure seamless communication and coordination among healthcare providers. They liaise with doctors, nurses, and other healthcare professionals to develop and implement comprehensive care plans tailored to patients' medical needs.

Nurse case managers often track patient outcomes through follow-up assessments and ensure compliance with treatment plans. They play a key role in identifying any complications or changes in patients' health status.

The nurse supports by providing additional education to patients about their conditions, treatment options, and self-management strategies. Nurse case managers advocate for the patient's medical needs within the healthcare system.

While their focus is more on the clinical aspects, nurse case managers also consider psychosocial factors and work collaboratively with social workers to address these needs.

5.2 Social Worker Role

The Social Worker brings a skill set that supports patients to achieve and maintain optimal health and wellness using a holistic approach.

Social workers emphasize the psychological, emotional, and social aspects of patient care. They assess the patient's social environment, mental health, and personal circumstances to identify any barriers to health and well-being.

The social worker provide counseling and support to patients and families, helping them cope with the emotional impact of illness. Social workers often facilitate support groups and connect patients with community resources.

Social workers help patients access external services such as financial assistance, transportation, or housing. They act as liaisons between patients and various social services or support organizations.

Social workers are instrumental in discharge planning, ensuring that patients have the necessary support systems in place before leaving the healthcare facility to meet the specific psychosocial needs and working with the nurse case manager to incorporate the medical needs for continued care and health management.

They often advocate for systemic changes within the healthcare system to address social determinants of health and improve patient access to care.

5.3 Collaboration Between Roles

Both nurse case managers and social workers collaborate closely to provide comprehensive care. While nurse case managers focus on the medical and clinical aspects of patient management, social workers address the psychosocial factors. Together, they enhance patient experience and outcomes by providing holistic support that includes both medical treatment and emotional well-being. Their teamwork fosters a multidisciplinary approach to case management, ensuring that patients receive well-rounded care throughout their healthcare journey.

The expanded role of Case Management reflects the evolving landscape of healthcare, emphasizing the importance of collaborative, patient-centered care. By effectively managing their responsibilities and coordinating with multiple stakeholders, Case Management teams can significantly enhance the quality of care and improve outcomes for patients during their entire continuum of care.

5.4 Supporting Patients Across the Continuum of Care

The Case Manager plays a crucial role in supporting patients across the continuum of care during hospitalization in several ways:

Upon admission, the Case Manager assesses the patient's needs, identifying any barriers to care, and develops a personalized care plan that addresses medical, social, and emotional needs. This is a required step as part of the Conditions of Participation.

They act as a liaison among the healthcare team, including doctors, nurses, and specialists, ensuring that everyone is on the same page regarding the patient's treatment and care plan. This coordination helps to minimize delays and improve patient outcomes.

The Case Manager provides education to the patient and their family about the treatment process, discharge plans, medications, and any necessary follow-up care. This education empowers patients to take an active role in their recovery.

They help patients access resources such as physical therapy, home health care, or community resources that may be needed post-discharge, ensuring a smooth transition from hospital to home or other care settings.

The Case Manager leads the discharge planning process, considering the patient's medical condition and social circumstances. This includes ensuring that there is a follow-up plan in place and that any necessary services or support are arranged beforehand.

After discharge, the Case Manager may continue to monitor the patient's progress through follow-up calls or appointments, helping manage any complications and ensuring continuity of care.

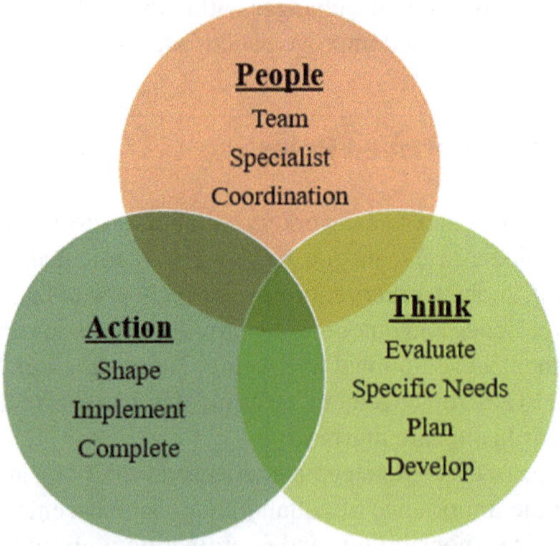

Fig. 5.1 The three key elements in provide quality care are people, think and action alignment. Created by the author

By fulfilling these roles, Case Managers ensure that patients receive comprehensive support throughout their hospital stay and beyond, ultimately leading to better health outcomes and improved patient satisfaction (Fig. 5.1).

5.5 Discharge Planning

One of the foundational roles of Case Management is to ensure that patients are discharged from the hospital in a timely and safe manner. This critical function requires collaboration among healthcare professionals, patients, and their families to create a seamless transition from institutional care to home or other care settings. It is essential for the Case Management team to adopt a holistic approach that takes into account not only the clinical aspects of a patient's health but also their emotional, social, and economic realities.

The Case Management team conducts thorough assessments of each patient's situation, identifying potential barriers that might impede a successful discharge. These barriers can range from medical needs and social circumstances to financial constraints and lack of support at home. For instance, patients suffering from chronic illnesses may require ongoing treatment or specialized care that isn't readily available outside the hospital. By recognizing these challenges early in the process, the team can develop a tailored discharge plan that addresses individual patient needs and preferences.

As part of this planning, Case Managers coordinate essential services and connect patients with necessary resources. This may involve arranging for home health services, acquiring medical equipment, or organizing follow-up medical appointments. It is equally important for the Case Management team to set realistic expectations for patients and their families regarding recovery timelines and potential risks associated with their conditions. Education plays a vital role in this process; patients and their families are informed about medications, recovery expectations, and potentially critical signs that require medical attention. Such awareness empowers patients to take an active role in their recovery.

While discharge planning is a crucial component of case management, it also reflects compliance with the Conditions of Participation set forth by regulatory bodies. Standardizing discharge processes not only enhances patient safety and satisfaction but also ensures that the healthcare facility meets required compliance standards. This dual focus on safety and compliance helps cultivate an environment where quality care can flourish.

Implementing evidence-based practices and continuous quality improvement initiatives, Case Management teams can significantly reduce readmission rates and foster better health outcomes for patients. This is particularly important, as frequent readmissions can be indicative of gaps in care or insufficient discharge planning. An effective discharge plan, therefore, is not just about facilitating a smooth transition out of the hospital; it is fundamentally about safeguarding the long-term health and well-being of patients post-discharge.

In addition to these logistical and clinical aspects, the emotional support provided during discharge planning cannot be underestimated. Transitioning from hospital

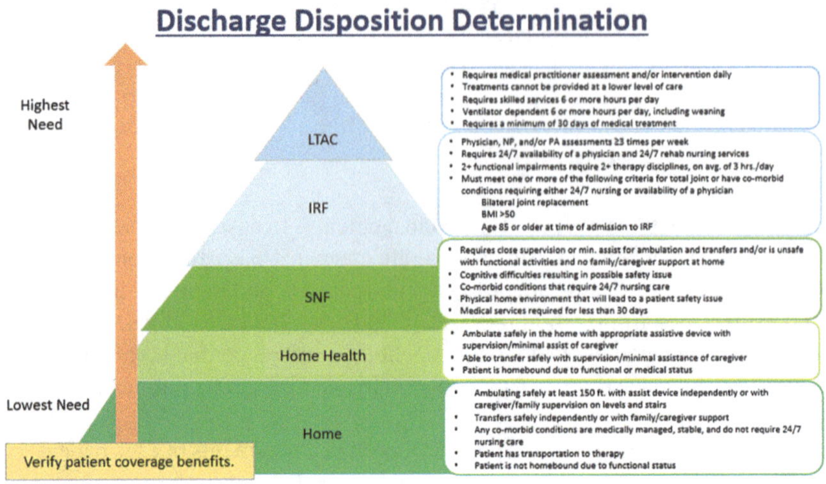

Fig. 5.2 Use CMS guidelines to determine the correct level of post-acute care supports patient return to optimal health. Created by the author

care can be daunting for many patients, and having a dedicated Case Manager who advocates for their needs and addresses their concerns can ease anxiety. The Case Management team's commitment to patient-centered care actively contributes to a smoother transition and overall continuity of care. By fostering open lines of communication, encouraging questions, and involving patients in decision-making, Case Managers help to build trust and promote positive experiences throughout the discharge process. This comprehensive approach ultimately serves to enhance the quality of care provided, ensuring that patients are not just leaving the hospital, but are better prepared and supported in their journey toward recovery (Fig. 5.2).

5.6 Care Coordination

Case Management plays a vital role in supporting patients as they navigate the often-complex landscape of the healthcare system. One of the primary responsibilities of Case Managers is to assist patients in understanding their health insurance coverage. This means helping them interpret policy details, educating them about benefits, including preventive services, and clarifying any potential out-of-pocket costs they might face. By demystifying health insurance terms and conditions, Case Managers empower patients to make informed decisions about their care and financial obligations.

In addition to insurance guidance, Case Managers act as a vital link, connecting patients with appropriate healthcare providers who can address their specific medical needs. This involves not only identifying the right specialists or primary care physicians but also ensuring that patients have the necessary referrals and that they understand how to prepare for their appointments. Preparation can include discussing what questions to ask, understanding the importance of following through with recommended tests or procedures, and providing tips on how to communicate effectively with healthcare providers.

Advocacy is another key component of Case Management. Case Managers work diligently to ensure that patients' voices are heard within the healthcare system. This may involve communicating with doctors and healthcare facilities to express patient needs, preferences, and concerns, thereby fostering a more patient-centered approach to care. This advocacy extends beyond immediate medical needs; it can also encompass emotional and psychological support, helping patients navigate their feelings about their health condition and treatment options.

The Case Management team is dedicated to ensuring that patients receive care that is both appropriate and cost-effective. They strategize to avoid unnecessary hospitalizations and readmissions by coordinating follow-up care, providing education on self-management strategies, and facilitating access to community resources. These resources may include support groups, counseling services, or local health initiatives, which further bolster the patient's overall well-being.

Case Managers often collaborate with multidisciplinary teams, comprising nurses, social workers, and other healthcare professionals, to create a comprehensive care plan tailored to each patient's unique situation. By maintaining open lines of communication among all parties involved in a patient's care, they help to streamline processes and reduce the likelihood of miscommunication or errors.

In essence, Case Management serves as a crucial support system for patients, guiding them through their healthcare journeys to achieve the best possible health outcomes while effectively navigating various challenges. This holistic approach not only addresses immediate medical concerns but also fosters long-term health and wellness, illustrating the indispensable value of Case Management in today's healthcare environment.

5.7 Readmission Risk Management

The Center for Medicare and Medicaid Services (CMS) has taken an important step towards improving healthcare quality by implementing a national reporting standard focused on readmission data. This initiative is vital for enhancing quality measures and creating transparent rating systems that are accessible to the public. By addressing readmission rates, healthcare providers can ensure that patients receive the highest standard of care, which is crucial for fostering trust in the healthcare system.

Effective care coordination plays a critical role in this effort, as it allows healthcare teams to identify patients who are at a higher risk of being readmitted to the hospital or making repeat visits to the emergency department. Standardizing the identification process and implementing timely and appropriate interventions is essential for developing a robust readmission prevention program that meets patient needs efficiently.

To achieve meaningful outcomes, it is necessary to systematically identify patients who have experienced readmissions. This involves conducting a thorough assessment of the underlying causes that led to their return. By understanding these root causes, healthcare providers can confirm that they have been effectively addressed before the patient is discharged. This proactive approach not only involves clinicians but also actively engages patients and their families in care planning, promoting a sense of responsibility and empowerment in managing health conditions.

Interventions can then be strategically established during the patient's stay. These could range from enhancing patient education about their condition and treatment plans to setting up follow-up appointments or home healthcare services post-discharge. Implementing these measures not only helps to prevent readmissions but also promotes better health outcomes, improves patient satisfaction, and reduces healthcare costs, ultimately contributing to a more efficient healthcare system.

By adopting a standardized approach to identifying at-risk patients and addressing their needs, the healthcare system can significantly reduce readmission rates. This, in turn, contributes to a healthier population and more sustainable healthcare practices. Such a comprehensive strategy positions healthcare providers to improve not only the quality of care but also the efficiency of healthcare delivery over time, ensuring that patients receive the support necessary for long-term health and recovery.

5.8 Readmission Risk Mitigation

Identifying patients at risk of readmission or repeat Emergency Department (ED) visits is a critical aspect of effective healthcare management. This identification process entails a thorough evaluation of various risk factors, including the patient's medical history, social determinants of health, and existing comorbidities. Understanding the factors that contribute to these risks not only empowers healthcare professionals to implement targeted interventions before patients are discharged, but also improves the planning of post-discharge care protocols. By proactively addressing potential complications or barriers to recovery—such as inadequate follow-up care or limited access to necessary medications—we can significantly mitigate the likelihood of readmission or unnecessary return visits to the ED (Fig. 5.3).

This holistic and proactive approach not only enhances patient outcomes but also contributes to the more efficient use of healthcare resources, thus alleviating pressure on the system. In an era where patient-centered care is paramount, refining our strategies to identify at-risk individuals can lead to improved health trajectories. Additionally, implementing education and support for both patients and their families plays a vital role in recovery, as it equips them with the necessary tools and knowledge. Ultimately, this concerted effort leads to a reduction in healthcare costs and fosters a healthier community overall, promoting well-being for all individuals and ensuring that healthcare systems can better focus on preventive care and long-term health solutions (Fig. 5.3).

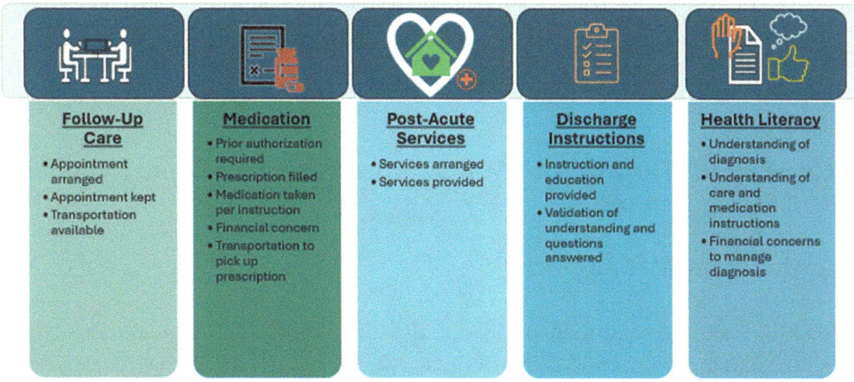

Fig. 5.3 Identify the root cause of readmission using a structured review of the 5 most common impacting factors. Created by the author

5.9 Readmission Assessment After Readmission

Once a patient has been readmitted or has returned to the Emergency Department, it is essential for the Case Manager to engage with the patient and their family in a thorough and compassionate manner. This meeting should aim to explore the underlying causes of the readmission or repeat visit in detail, fostering an open dialogue that encourages patients and their families to share their experiences and concerns. Understanding the specific factors that led to this situation—whether related to the patient's medical condition, lack of support systems, or challenges in adhering to post-discharge instructions—can provide invaluable insights that drive meaningful change.

Armed with this information, healthcare facilities can take significant steps toward process improvements that directly address the reasons for readmission. For instance, they can develop more tailored discharge plans that accommodate the unique needs of high-risk patients, ensuring they leave the hospital equipped with the necessary resources, knowledge, and support. Establishing partnerships with community organizations and external healthcare providers can greatly enhance the continuum of care, providing robust support systems for patients after discharge. This includes offering access to follow-up care, medication management, mental health services, and home health services, all of which play a crucial role in ensuring that patients do not return to the hospital unnecessarily.

Additionally, evaluating the data collected from readmissions is vital for identifying trends and patterns that may indicate systemic issues within the healthcare system. This analysis allows for larger-scale changes to be implemented, targeting the root causes of readmissions rather than just the symptoms. Such a proactive approach can lead to the development of new services and educational programs designed to equip patients and their families with the tools and knowledge they need to manage their health effectively and independently.

Employing a comprehensive strategy that includes pre-discharge assessments, thorough post-readmission evaluations, and collaboration with community resources can drastically reduce the rates of readmission and repeat visits to the Emergency Department. By focusing on improved communication, patient education, and establishing support networks, healthcare facilities can ensure that patients feel empowered in their healthcare journey. Ultimately, through this commitment to improving patient care and fostering a supportive environment, healthcare facilities can enhance patient satisfaction and outcomes, while also promoting overall efficacy in managing healthcare resources and reducing healthcare costs.

5.10 Patient Throughput Management and Bed Capacity Management

Length of Stay Management

In the healthcare sector, effective care coordination is essential for guaranteeing that patients receive the appropriate level of care while optimizing the use of available resources. This process encompasses a variety of elements including communication, resource allocation, and strategic planning. To achieve optimal outcomes, establishing a systematic process for case reviews and information sharing among the care team is critical. Such a collaborative approach not only enhances the team's collective understanding of the patient's needs, medical history, and treatment plan but ultimately contributes to delivering high-quality and holistic care.

According to the New England Journal of Medicine, each day a patient spends in a hospital carries an approximate 1% risk of developing a hospital-acquired infection (HAI). Therefore, managing the length of a patient's hospital stay goes beyond mere logistics; it has profound implications for patient safety. It not only has the potential to reduce the risk of HAI but also plays a crucial role in enhancing patient outcomes. Effective care coordination aids in smooth transitions between different stages of care, significantly diminishing unnecessary delays and complications. By ensuring that all members of the healthcare team are aligned and informed, we can mitigate risks and improve overall service delivery.

In recent years, the management of patient throughput and bed capacity has garnered increasing attention within case management. As the healthcare landscape evolves, heavily influenced by technological advancements and changing patient demographics, the demand for efficient and timely care has made it essential to re-evaluate and optimize processes related to patient movement through the healthcare system. This is where a robust focus on care coordination becomes indispensable. It ensures that patients receive timely interventions and facilitates an environment where they are moved seamlessly from admission to discharge.

In a coordinated care model, healthcare providers, including physicians, nurses, social workers, therapists, and other specialists, work collaboratively to address all aspects of a patient's needs. This teamwork not only helps streamline care delivery but also enhances patient satisfaction by ensuring that patients feel heard, informed, and actively involved in their treatment plans. Engaging patients in their own care is increasingly recognized as an essential component of successful treatment; it empowers them and can lead to increased adherence to prescribed therapies.

By focusing on effective communication and the sharing of vital information across the care continuum, healthcare professionals can better anticipate and respond to the evolving needs of their patients. Regular interdisciplinary team meetings, shared electronic health records, and defined communication protocols serve as mechanisms to facilitate this critical information sharing, ensuring that everyone involved in the patient's care is on the same page.

Establishing a basic workflow for managing all aspects of patient care is not merely an operational necessity; it serves as a foundational pillar for overall throughput management. Processes that standardize care, eliminate redundancies, and facilitate timely decision-making empower teams to deliver care that is not only efficient but also compassionate and responsive to each patient's unique circumstances.

Additionally, the integration of data analytics and technology can provide valuable insights that guide decision-making and process improvements. Tracking key performance indicators (KPI) allows for the identification of bottlenecks and areas for improvement, which can be instrumental in achieving system-wide efficiencies.

Overall, the overarching goal of improved care coordination is to achieve better health outcomes, reduce the risk of complications, and ultimately enhance the quality of life for patients within the healthcare system. By prioritizing care coordination, we can ensure that the healthcare system functions more effectively, leading to satisfied patients and healthier communities.

Length of Stay Outlier Management

Effective management of patient throughput and bed capacity is paramount for healthcare facilities aiming to deliver high-quality care. As patients increasingly present for medical attention at more advanced stages of their illnesses or with multiple coexisting conditions, they may experience prolonged hospital stays that exceed typical expectations. This scenario not only strains hospital resources but also poses significant challenges for care coordination, impacting the overall efficiency of healthcare delivery.

To mitigate these growing issues, early identification and timely intervention are essential components. It is critical for healthcare providers to proactively assess patients at risk of extended stays, ensuring that they can implement targeted interventions that facilitate smoother transitions of care. Such an approach enables hospital beds to remain available for incoming patients from various entry points, effectively reducing backlogs in Emergency Departments and minimizing delays in care delivery.

To tackle the complexities associated with managing length of stay, healthcare organizations can consider establishing dedicated length-of-stay management teams. Alternatively, organizations may enhance the existing Care Coordination team by incorporating specialized processes aimed at addressing these challenges. This dedicated team can focus on evaluating patient cases that are likely to lead to extended hospitalizations, actively implementing targeted strategies to improve patient flow, and enhancing communication among the multidisciplinary care team involved in patient management.

Once these processes are in place and operating effectively, healthcare facilities can anticipate a noticeable decrease in the length of stay for complex cases. Successful interventions can become integrated into the daily functions of the Care Coordination team, establishing a culture of continuous improvement within the organization. This proactive approach not only optimizes resource utilization, but also significantly enhances the overall patient experience. Healthcare providers can ensure that each patient receives timely and appropriate care, ultimately supporting better health outcomes and operational efficiency within the healthcare system.

By prioritizing patient throughput and strategically leveraging organizational changes, healthcare facilities can navigate the challenges posed by increasingly complex patient needs. In doing so, they maintain a steadfast commitment to patient-centered care, which is essential in today's rapidly evolving healthcare landscape. This commitment ensures that patients receive the quality of care they deserve while also allowing healthcare organizations to function effectively in the face of rising demand. Ultimately, these measures can lead to a more resilient healthcare system that is better equipped to meet future challenges.

High-Risk for Length of Stay Outlier Identification

Identifying patients at risk for extended hospital stays exemplifies the essential collaboration between the Utilization Review, Clinical Documentation Integrity, and Case Management departments. Each of these departments possesses vital information that can significantly impact patient care and hospital efficiency.

Utilization Review plays a key role in assessing the medical necessity and appropriateness of hospital admissions and continued stays. By analyzing patient data and treatment plans, this department can identify potential barriers to discharge and highlight cases that may require additional resources or interventions. This proactive assessment not only helps in minimizing unnecessary stays but also promotes a more streamlined admission process, directly affecting overall hospital throughput.

Similarly, the Clinical Documentation Integrity team ensures that patient records accurately reflect the severity of illness and the complexity of care provided. Comprehensive and precise documentation is critical, as it not only supports appropriate reimbursement but also informs the care team about the patient's specific needs, thereby facilitating more effective planning and resource allocation. A well-documented record can also foster better communication across care teams, which is pivotal for a successful discharge process.

Case Management acts as the bridge between these processes, coordinating care and resources to ensure patients receive the appropriate services at the right time. By engaging with patients, families, and healthcare providers, Case Management can address social determinants of health, coordinate post-discharge care, and identify necessary follow-up services. This interaction often highlights underlying issues that may delay discharge, such as lack of home care or necessary equipment.

Bringing these departments together fosters a holistic approach to patient care, enabling the healthcare team to proactively manage cases that may otherwise lead to prolonged hospital stays. Such collaboration not only enhances patient outcomes but also optimizes hospital operations, reduces costs, and improves overall patient satisfaction. By leveraging each department's distinct strengths and insights, we can create a more integrated and effective care delivery model, ultimately benefiting both patients and healthcare providers alike, and paving the way for continuous improvement in quality of care across the healthcare system.

Length of Stay Outlier High-Level Management

The early identification and management of patients who may be at risk of becoming outliers in terms of length of stay is crucial for optimizing both patient care and the efficient use of healthcare resources. Addressing this issue effectively can significantly improve patient outcomes while also ensuring that healthcare facilities operate at maximum efficiency. A collaborative, team-based approach is essential in this process, as it ensures that various aspects of patient care are addressed comprehensively and holistically.

Case Managers (CM) play a pivotal role by identifying social determinants of health that could contribute to a patient's risk factors. These may include elements such as socioeconomic status, access to transportation, housing stability, and support systems, which can significantly affect a patient's recovery process and length of stay. By recognizing these factors early, CMs can initiate targeted interventions that may help mitigate potential delays in discharge and facilitate smoother transitions to post-acute care settings or home.

Similarly, Utilization Management (UM) professionals are tasked with identifying medical necessity risks that could impact a patient's care. They assess the appropriateness of treatments and interventions to ensure that patients receive the right level of care at the right time. This assessment process is not merely about rationing services, but it is also about effectively coordinating the patient's care pathway, ensuring that interventions are both necessary and beneficial. By monitoring these aspects closely, UM can help prevent unnecessary extended hospital stays that may arise from mismanagement or overutilization of services. Additionally, proactive engagement with healthcare providers can enhance compliance with clinical guidelines.

The Clinical Documentation Integrity (CDI) specialists play a critical role by identifying potential Diagnosis-Related Groups (DRG) that might indicate a higher likelihood of longer hospital stays. Accurate and thorough documentation ensures that patients are classified correctly, which is essential for appropriate reimbursement and resource allocation. Detecting potential DRG issues early allows for timely interventions that can improve clinical outcomes and significantly reduce length of stay. The clarity and precision in documentation also contribute to data accuracy that can influence hospital quality scores and metrics.

By escalating cases that show risks for prolonged hospitalization to the multidisciplinary team early in the process, healthcare professionals can collaboratively develop targeted strategies for each patient. This proactive management approach not only enhances patient outcomes but also contributes to the overall efficiency of the healthcare facility. By working together, CM, UM, and CDI professionals can create a holistic management plan that addresses both the clinical and social needs of patients. This collaborative effort ultimately leads to improved resource utilization and patient satisfaction, creating a more patient-centered environment where healthcare delivery is both effective and compassionate. It is through this synergy that healthcare teams can ensure that patients receive not only the best of medical care but also the support necessary to thrive in their recovery journeys.

Long Stay Management of Custodial Cases

As the population ages, the demand for long-term care services continues to rise significantly. This increasing demand places considerable pressure on hospitals, which are often called upon to fulfill the role of providing this essential care. However, it is important to recognize that not all patients require hospital-level treatment. Many individuals may need assistance with daily activities but do not necessitate the intensive medical interventions typically associated with hospital care. This distinction is crucial for optimizing healthcare resources and ensuring that patients receive the most appropriate level of care tailored to their unique situations.

Alongside the growing demand for long-term care, the complexity of individual patient needs is becoming more apparent. Many patients face a variety of barriers that prevent them from returning to their previous living situations after hospitalization. Safety concerns arise due to physical impairments, cognitive decline, or a lack of supportive resources at home. These factors can greatly complicate the reintegration process back into the community after hospitalization. For some, the home environment may pose risks that make it unsafe for them to live independently. With declining health, the need for a structured and secure living arrangement becomes essential to prevent further health deterioration or accidents.

This situation creates a complex dilemma for case managers, who are tasked with facilitating the discharge process for patients. It is not merely a matter of following protocols; rather, case managers must navigate the delicate balance of ensuring that patients receive appropriate care while also adhering to discharge protocols that emphasize medical necessity. This balancing act requires a profound understanding of the individual patient's circumstances, along with an awareness of the resources available within the community.

Case managers must advocate for alternative care options that align with the unique needs of each patient. These alternatives can include rehabilitation facilities, assisted living arrangements, or home health services, all of which can offer varying levels of support. By advocating for a personalized approach to care, case managers can significantly influence the trajectory of a patient's recovery and overall quality of life. It is essential for them to take a holistic view of the patient's situation, considering not only their medical conditions but also their social, emotional, and environmental factors.

In addition to advocating for proper care, case managers also work collaboratively with families, healthcare providers, and community resources. This collaborative approach is vital for creating safe and sustainable discharge plans that prioritize the well-being of patients while addressing the constraints of the healthcare system. Engaging families in the process can provide additional support and insights into the patient's needs and preferences, ensuring that the discharge plan is comprehensive and realistic.

Education plays a pivotal role in this process, as many families may not fully understand the resources available to them or the steps necessary for a successful transition from hospital to home or a different care facility. Case managers can provide essential information, empowering families to make informed decisions regarding their loved ones' care. This education can extend to the importance of follow-up care, community resources, and support systems that can help sustain a patient's health after discharge.

In this evolving landscape of healthcare, it's crucial to rethink our approaches to long-term care. By fostering communication, collaboration, and advocacy, stakeholders can work together to ensure that all patients are afforded the opportunity to recover in environments that support their safety and independence. Understanding that the path to recovery is not one-size-fits-all is essential in creating a future where healthcare is responsive and resilient, ultimately leading to improved outcomes for patients and families alike. Therefore, embracing innovative solutions and policies that adapt to the complexities of long-term care will be fundamental in addressing the pressing needs of an aging population in a compassionate and effective manner.

5.11 Avoidable Days and Delays

Excess days in the hospital—defined as the duration a patient remains admitted beyond the medically necessary timeframe—are a critical issue frequently discussed among healthcare executives and stakeholders within the industry. These excess days not only impact bed capacity but also significantly affect the financial health and operational efficiency of healthcare facilities. When patients remain in the hospital longer than necessary, it can lead to overcrowding, delayed admissions for new patients, and increased costs associated with staffing and resources required to care for them.

From a Care Coordination perspective, excess days are recognized as unnecessary prolongations of a patient's stay, which often stem from avoidable delays in care. These delays can have various root causes, including logistical challenges, staffing shortages, or communication gaps within the care team. Such avoidable days can hinder the timely delivery of care for other patients, ultimately affecting overall patient throughput and operational efficiency. Several studies demonstrate that long hospital stays can sometimes lead to complications, increasing the risk of infections and further health issues for patients.

To effectively manage resources and minimize these unnecessary delays, it is vital for facilities to implement a robust process dedicated to identifying and intervening in cases where avoidable days may occur. This effort requires proactive involvement from every member of the care team, including nursing staff, physicians, social workers, and case managers. The collaboration across departments is also essential; for instance, engaging with the admissions team, pharmacy, and rehabilitation services can help streamline processes and alleviate bottlenecks that contribute to extended hospital stays.

As highlighted in the section covering length of stay outliers, many cases within the facility are directly influenced by avoidable days and delays in care. While it's important to recognize that not every avoidable day can be controlled solely by care coordination or clinical teams, the data collected from these cases prove invaluable. This information can guide performance improvement initiatives and also serve as a foundation for meaningful discussions around contracting and partnerships with payors and other healthcare entities.

Tackling the issue of excess days requires a concerted effort from all stakeholders involved in patient care. By fostering a culture of accountability and continuous improvement, facilities can enhance the patient experience, maximize resource utilization, and ultimately drive better health outcomes for the communities they serve. Such a holistic approach not only benefits the patients by ensuring they receive appropriate care in a timely manner but also bolsters the healthcare system's ability to operate efficiently and sustainably.

5.12 Avoidable Days and Delays Cause-Specific

In healthcare and service delivery, understanding the factors that contribute to avoidable days and delays is crucial for enhancing patient outcomes and operational efficiency. These unnecessary extensions in patient stays or service timelines can often be traced back to common underlying issues that require close examination. By identifying and categorizing these root causes, we can develop targeted strategies to mitigate them effectively and improve overall service delivery.

This exploration aims to not only shed light on these challenges but also to provide a comprehensive framework for improving processes and ultimately ensuring a more streamlined experience for both patients and providers. By implementing these insights, organizations can foster an environment that prioritizes timely care while minimizing disruptions.

As we dive deeper into the standard root causes of avoidable days and delays, we will break them down into manageable categories for a clearer understanding. This categorization will allow healthcare professionals to focus their efforts on specific areas that need improvement, thus leading to enhanced patient experiences, reduced costs, and improved operational workflows. Ultimately, understanding these factors can lead to more responsive and effective healthcare systems that are better equipped to meet the needs of their patients.

Patient/Family Barriers

The barriers encountered in a patient's care and discharge planning frequently stem from the engagement levels of the patient and their family members. Effective communication and active participation are essential for successful care transitions. This engagement often hinges on the availability of family members or caregivers who can attend care conferences and actively participate in calls to discuss critical aspects of the patient's treatment, such as progress updates, adjustments to care goals, and the impacts of cognitive decline on decision-making capacities.

When family involvement is limited, it can lead to confusion and misalignment regarding the patient's needs and preferences, ultimately contributing to unnecessary hospital stays and delays in discharge. For instance, when family members are unaware of discharge plans or changes in treatment, the patient may not receive the necessary support at home to manage their recovery effectively. By enhancing care coordination processes and emphasizing early identification of potential barriers, many of these avoidable days in the hospital can be significantly minimized.

Collaboration with other departments, such as social work, rehabilitation, and mental health services, may be necessary to provide comprehensive support and resources tailored to the individual patient's needs. Implementing targeted strategies that foster family engagement and ensure a seamless flow of information among all stakeholders involved in the patient's care is crucial in achieving optimal patient outcomes. This may include regular updates, educational resources, and opportunities for family members to voice their concerns and questions.

Ultimately, addressing these barriers not only supports the patient's journey toward recovery but also empowers families to be active participants in the decision-making process, creating a more holistic approach to patient-centered care. By prioritizing family involvement, healthcare providers can enhance patient satisfaction and improve the overall quality of care delivered, leading to better health outcomes and a more supportive recovery environment.

Clinical Complex Care Cases

Managing patients with clinical complexity and unexpected complications presents significant challenges in healthcare settings. While it might be unavoidable to encounter such patients, it is essential to recognize that their multifaceted conditions often result in prolonged hospital stays, which can lead to increased healthcare costs, resource strain, and overwhelming demands on healthcare staff.

Effective care coordination efforts play a vital role in addressing these issues. By meticulously identifying, analyzing, and understanding the potential causes that contribute to extended care duration, healthcare teams can implement strategic interventions designed to streamline the care process. Common factors that may prolong a patient's stay include delays in revising treatment plans, the need for additional services, and the involvement of multiple providers, which can complicate the care process significantly.

Clinical teams dedicated to care coordination work proactively to manage these potentially avoidable hospitalization days and delays. Their tasks may involve streamlining communication among healthcare providers, ensuring timely updates to treatment plans, and facilitating prompt access to necessary services that patients require. Additionally, by engaging with patients and their families throughout the process, care coordinators can help clarify expectations, foster understanding, and collaborate effectively on discharge planning.

Ultimately, the goal is to enhance the overall patient experience while optimizing resource utilization within healthcare systems. Focusing on communication and collaborative efforts can make a profound difference. By targeting these areas, care coordination can significantly reduce the length of hospital stays for complex cases, improve overall patient outcomes, and create a more efficient healthcare delivery model that benefits everyone involved. This approach not only addresses immediate patient needs but also lays the groundwork for future healthcare improvements and innovations.

External Provider Barriers

Healthcare facilities increasingly depend on external and community providers to facilitate the ongoing care and treatment that patients require prior to their discharge. For example, before being able to return home, a patient might need access to skilled nursing facilities or acute rehabilitation services. Any delays in the assessment, determination, or acceptance of the required care can lead to prolonged hospital stays, which not only impact patient satisfaction but also strain hospital resources and increase operational costs.

While it is true that not all delays can be managed through effective care coordination or follow-up communications, a significant portion of these challenges can be addressed by delivering comprehensive data to facility leadership. This data serves a critical role in fostering discussions among healthcare professionals and making informed decisions about various care pathways. For healthcare facilities that are part of an Accountable Care Organization (ACO), such data becomes especially crucial. It enables leadership to evaluate partnership opportunities more effectively, identify strategies for enhancing the quality of care delivered by partner organizations, and improve overall patient outcomes.

By analyzing these delays and the related patient outcomes, facilities can develop targeted strategies aimed at reducing unnecessary extended hospital stays. Implementing robust data-sharing practices not only empowers leadership to make informed decisions but also ensures that care transitions are executed smoothly. This ultimately results in a more efficient healthcare system that prioritizes patient-centered care. Such a proactive approach not only supports the health and well-being of patients but also aligns with the broader goals of improving healthcare quality, enhancing patient experiences, and reducing costs across the entire continuum of care. By addressing these barriers effectively, healthcare facilities can contribute to a more cohesive and responsive healthcare environment.

Internal/System Barriers

Care coordination processes play a pivotal role in enhancing the efficiency and effectiveness of healthcare delivery, particularly when it comes to minimizing avoidable days and delays within the healthcare system. Effective care coordination not only streamlines patient care but also ensures that all team members are aligned and informed about a patient's needs and progress, which ultimately contributes to improved health outcomes. To reduce potential delays, it is crucial to foster an environment where patient needs are thoroughly discussed during treatment team meetings. These discussions should not merely be routine but should focus on identifying specific challenges, barriers, and resources required for each patient's unique situation.

Appointing a dedicated individual to facilitate these meetings can significantly enhance the prioritization and execution of necessary services. This facilitator's role should include tracking the implementation of care plans, ensuring that all team members are actively contributing, and diligently following up on outstanding tasks to prevent potential issues from escalating. The collection and analysis of data pertaining to care coordination can unveil critical insights into the potential requirements for increased staffing levels, extended hours of service coverage, or the introduction of new services that may be beneficial for patient management. By identifying trends and patterns in patient care, leadership teams can make informed decisions that align with strategic planning and budgeting processes.

Engaging frontline staff in this analysis not only bolsters team morale but also encourages input from those who are directly involved in patient care. The insights gained from this data can help not only in optimizing resource allocation but also in enhancing overall patient outcomes and satisfaction. By prioritizing effective care coordination and utilizing data-driven insights, healthcare systems can create a more responsive and patient-centered environment that reduces avoidable delays and fosters better health outcomes for all patients, ultimately leading to a more resilient healthcare system overall.

Payor Barriers

The data regarding avoidable days and delays related to payors primarily focuses on the authorization process necessary for transitioning to the next level of care or for providing specific services. This authorization process can often be complex and subject to various regulations, which complicates matters for healthcare providers and patients alike. Consequently, it becomes essential for the Case Manager to actively engage in consistent communication with the payors, making persistent calls and follow-ups to secure the necessary authorization.

In doing so, the Case Manager must harness strong interpersonal skills to advocate effectively for the patient's needs. This proactive approach not only involves navigating intricate bureaucratic processes but also requires the Case Manager to stay informed about payor policies and guidelines that may vary significantly. By effectively overcoming these challenges, the Case Manager plays a crucial role in minimizing delays and ensuring that patients receive timely and appropriate care that is crucial for their recovery.

Due diligence in communication and authorization not only helps in reducing avoidable days but also enhances the overall efficiency of the care delivery process. In essence, when Case Managers prioritize these efforts, they contribute to better health outcomes, improved patient satisfaction, and optimized resource use within the healthcare system. The effectiveness of this role cannot be underestimated, as timely interventions are often critical in a patient's treatment journey.

Provider Barriers

This category focuses on identifying avoidable delays and additional patient days that necessitate thorough review and analysis. To effectively manage these situations, it is considered best practice to involve key figures such as a Physician Advisor, a Utilization Review provider, or a Chief Medical Officer (CMO). Their expertise is crucial in evaluating whether a specific provider contributed to the delay and determining the appropriate attribution for it.

The process can be quite complex within a hospital setting, particularly due to the nature of rotating coverage among providers. This situation often complicates accountability, as it may not necessarily be the provider of record who is responsible for the delay being assessed. In many cases, multiple providers may be involved in patient care, which reinforces the importance of a collaborative approach when examining the circumstances surrounding each case to ensure that all factors are duly considered.

An important note regarding the data relating to provider-specific avoidable delays and additional patient days is that this information is systematically compiled and forwarded to the Medical Staffing department for analysis. This information plays a vital role in the ongoing assessment of healthcare providers' performance and is instrumental in their inclusion in the annual Ongoing Professional Performance Evaluation (OPPE) process. By meticulously evaluating and analyzing these avoidable delays, healthcare organizations can enhance their operational efficiency, ultimately leading to improved patient care and satisfaction. Understanding the nuances behind these delays can shed light on areas needing improvement, allowing for targeted interventions and education for providers. This strategic focus can create a culture of accountability and continuous improvement that benefits both patients and healthcare staff alike.

5.13 Patient Care Rounds

Patient throughput management plays a crucial role in enhancing the overall quality of healthcare delivery. One of its key components is the implementation of treatment team rounds, which are designed to foster effective collaboration among healthcare professionals across various disciplines. These rounds not only aim to optimize patient care but also to ensure the efficient utilization of health service resources. By creating a coordinated and structured approach to patient care, treatment team rounds can significantly improve patient outcomes while streamlining the throughput processes within healthcare facilities.

Treatment team rounds are known by various names across different medical institutions, including Multidisciplinary Rounds (MDR), Interdisciplinary Team (IDT) meetings, Comprehensive Care Rounds (CCR), Multidisciplinary Care Conference (MCC), Structured Interdisciplinary Bedside Rounds (SIBR), Interprofessional Rounds (IR), and Patient Progression Rounds (PPR) and some of the examples. Regardless of the terminology used, the underlying principle remains the same: a comprehensive team of healthcare professionals from diverse fields gathers to collaboratively address the individual needs of each patient. This collaborative approach allows for a holistic

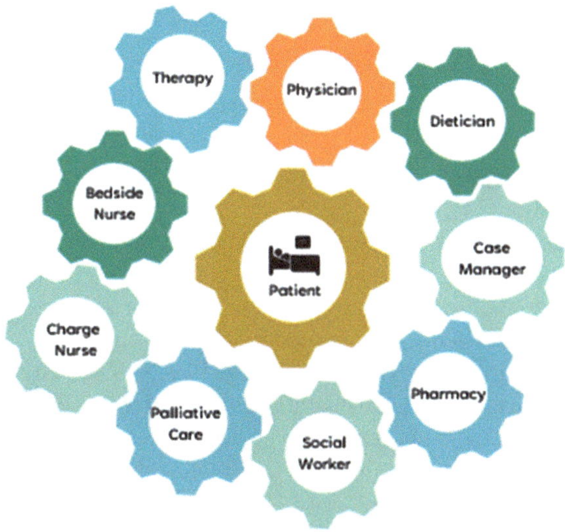

Fig. 5.4 A patient-centered approach to multidisciplinary healthcare supports consistency with communication and care. Created by the author

understanding of the patient's condition, ensuring that all aspects of care, including medical, psychological, and social factors, are taken into consideration (Fig. 5.4).

Establishing daily rounds for every unit in a healthcare facility is a crucial best practice that leads to significant improvements in patient care. These rounds ensure that all team members—physicians, nurses, pharmacists, social workers, and other specialists—are equipped with the latest and most relevant information concerning each patient's situation. This shared knowledge empowers the team to make informed decisions quickly and facilitates timely interventions and adjustments to care plans. Additionally, daily rounds promote continuity of care, enhance communication among departments, and reinforce a culture of teamwork and accountability.

Overall, the integration of treatment team rounds into patient throughput management is essential for achieving high-quality medical care. By promoting collaboration, enhancing communication, and streamlining processes, these rounds contribute to a holistic approach that ultimately benefits patients and improves the efficiency of healthcare systems. Emphasizing the importance of collective effort can lead to improved patient satisfaction, better health outcomes, and a more effective use of resources within the healthcare environment, ultimately enhancing the entire patient experience.

Example agendas for Medical/Surgical and ICU rounding Fig. 5.4:

5.14 Daily Rounds on Medical/Surgical Units

Attendees (at a minimum):

- Hospitalists
- Case Management Lead (facilitator)
- Care Coordinator/Social Work

- Nursing Representatives
- Therapy (PT, ST, OT)
- With a communication pathway for UR/CDI (via CC), RT/Pharmacy/Nutrition (via nursing)

Review/Discussion Priorities/Targets/Barriers
- Care Coordination
- Any new issues overnight or concerns from patient/family
- Needs for today (testing, evaluation, treatment) PLAN FOR THE DAY
- Avoidable Days and Barriers to discharge delays (CM to enter in the appropriate area of the patient's chart for data extraction)
- Goals needed to meet to be ready to discharge PLAN FOR THE STAY
- Target discharge date—enter into the patient's medical record PLAN TO GO AWAY
- Discharge plan, including backup if the first option is not working timely
  - Move D/C planning efforts ahead; no D/C's today should be a surprise or waiting on CM/SW
- ANY TEAM MEMBER: Enter templated documentation into the patient medical record (assign team member per unit determination – CM, SW, RN, other)
  - Billing for rounds is acceptable in some situations.

5.15 Daily Rounds for Intensive Care Units

Attendees:
- Hospitalists/Residents/Attending
- Case Manager (facilitator)
- Social Work
- Nursing Representatives
- RT (may be shared via nursing)
- Pharmacy (may be shared via nursing)
- Therapy (may be shared via nursing)
- With a communication pathway for UR for auth status/CDI for working DRG and GMLOS

Review/Discussion Priorities/Targets/Barriers
- Medical progression
  - Time of intubation
    - Time for transition to trach
  - Weaning
  - Time and output of chest tubes/drains
    - Goal for removal
  - Weaning IV medications
  - Sedation vacation

  - Bundle compliance
    - Central line
    - Ventilator
    - Sepsis
    - Oral care
    - Drain/catheter output and removal readiness
  - DVT prevention
  - GI stress prevention
  - Skin assessments
- Appropriate to transition to another unit/post-acute level of care with a goal date
- Goals of care changes
- Advance directives/POA
- Patient/family involvement in care
- Follow-up on previously identified issues
  - ANY TEAM MEMBER: Enter templated documentation into the patient medical record (assign team member per unit determination CM, SW, RN, other)
  - Documentation should not repeat documentation rather focus on discussion without mention of avoidable delays/days outside of the specified area in the HER.
  - Billing for rounds are acceptable in some situations.
- Identify any cases for appropriate escalation for length of stay outlier management
- Goal date of discharge from hospital (EDD)

By adhering to this structured approach, healthcare teams can ensure the highest standards and quality of care for their patients.

5.16 Discharge Care Team Huddles

Effective communication between nursing staff and Case Management is essential for optimizing patient care and ensuring smooth throughput in healthcare settings. To facilitate this, establishing a brief but focused rapid discharge huddle between the unit charge nurse and the Case Manager or Social Worker can significantly enhance collaboration and efficiency. These huddles, ideally lasting no more than five minutes, are designed to share critical information that can be utilized throughout the day.

The primary objective of these huddles is to align both teams with the current status of patient discharges, upcoming needs, and any potential barriers that might arise. By dedicating this time to discussing key aspects of patient care, the nursing staff and Case Management can more effectively manage their workloads, streamline daily operations, and proactively prepare for the following day.

Here are some essential topics that should be covered during these huddles:

Current Patient Status: Quick updates on patients scheduled for discharge, including any last-minute requirements or changes in their conditions that may affect their readiness for leaving the hospital and support a change in level of care status.

Anticipated Discharges: A review of which patients are expected to be discharged that day. This allows both teams to prepare accordingly and allocate resources efficiently to ensure a smooth transition for the patient.

Pending Tasks: Identification of any outstanding tasks related to patient care, such as the completion of discharge paperwork, securing follow-up appointments, or managing medication regimens. This ensures that no critical tasks are overlooked, which could potentially delay discharges.

Barriers to Discharge: Discuss any potential obstacles that could delay patient discharges—such as waiting for test results, consultations, or insurance authorizations—and strategize solutions to address them proactively. This step is crucial in maintaining the flow of patient care.

Patient Education Needs: Determine if patients require additional education or support before discharge, enabling Case Management to arrange necessary resources or referrals. Empowering patients with knowledge prior to their discharge can lead to better post-hospital outcomes.

Coordination of Resources: Share information about available community resources or services that may assist patients post-discharge, including home health options, rehabilitation services, or transportation assistance to help them transition smoothly back into their daily lives.

By incorporating these elements into the rapid discharge huddles, both the nursing staff and Case Management can foster a more integrated approach to patient care. This approach serves not only to improve safety and satisfaction but also enhances outcomes for patients.

The importance of regular, efficient communication cannot be overstated. It not merely aids in day-to-day operations but also builds a collaborative culture within the healthcare team. This culture of collaboration is vital for addressing any issues that arise during patient care, ultimately aiming for the highest standards in patient service delivery.

Rapid CM/Charge Nurse 0730 AM daily huddle:

The discharge (DC) process was held the prior day. What were the challenges encountered? Share any changes in patient condition with the Utilization Review (UR) team that could impact future discharges.

Identify which patients are expected to be discharged that same day to confirm readiness and plans for follow-up care.

Rapid CM/Charge Nurse 1530 PM daily huddle:

Discuss any discharges expected during the evening/night, ensuring that staff are prepared for any last-minute needs.

Review anticipated discharges for the following day and confirm that all teams are aligned on plans to facilitate these transitions smoothly.

These huddles are instrumental in keeping communication channels open and ensuring that patient care remains the top priority.

5.17 Transitional Care (TC) and Population Health

Case Managers play a crucial role in the continuum of healthcare services, ensuring that patients transition smoothly from one care setting to another. This period between hospital discharge and home care is often fraught with potential risks, such as medication errors, lack of follow-up care, and misunderstandings about treatment plans. Transitional Care Management (TCM) and Population Health (PH) aim to address these challenges by providing a structured and supportive framework for patients during this vulnerable time.

Case managers are at the heart of Transitional Care and Population Health, helping to create individualized care plans that cater to the specific needs of each patient. They work closely with healthcare providers, patients, and their families to ensure that all aspects of the patient's care are coordinated effectively. This includes arranging follow-up appointments, coordinating with primary care physicians and specialists, and ensuring that patients have access to necessary medications and medical equipment.

Transitional Care and Population Health programs often incorporate educational components to empower patients with the knowledge needed to manage their health independently. This education includes detailed explanations of their medical conditions, the importance of adhering to prescribed treatment regimens, and recognizing symptoms that may indicate complications. By providing patients with this information, case managers help to reduce the likelihood of readmissions and enhance patients' confidence in managing their own health.

In addition to direct patient care, Transitional Care and Population Health also encompasses the involvement of community resources and support systems. Case managers may connect patients with local organizations that offer additional assistance, such as transportation services, nutritional counseling, and mental health support. The integration of these resources into the care plan further bolsters the patient's ability to recover and thrive in their home environment. The expansion of access to Transitional Care and Population Health Management programs is essential for advancing patient outcomes and curbing rising healthcare costs. By increasing the availability of these programs, healthcare providers can facilitate better management of chronic conditions and complex health issues, ensuring patients have the necessary support as they navigate the healthcare landscape.

The importance of Transitional Care and Population Health is underscored by its ability to improve patient outcomes and generate cost savings for the healthcare system. Studies have shown that effective TCM and Population Health programs can lead to lower readmission rates, better management of chronic diseases, and higher patient satisfaction. Healthcare facilities benefit from reduced strain on hospital resources and more efficient use of staff time, while payors see a reduction in overall healthcare expenditures.

Transitional Care and Population Health Management is not just a bridge between hospital and home; it is a comprehensive approach that aims to optimize every aspect of patient care during a critical period. By focusing on personalized care plans, education, and community support, TCM programs create a robust safety net for patients, ensuring that they receive the right care at the right time. This patient-centered approach is essential for

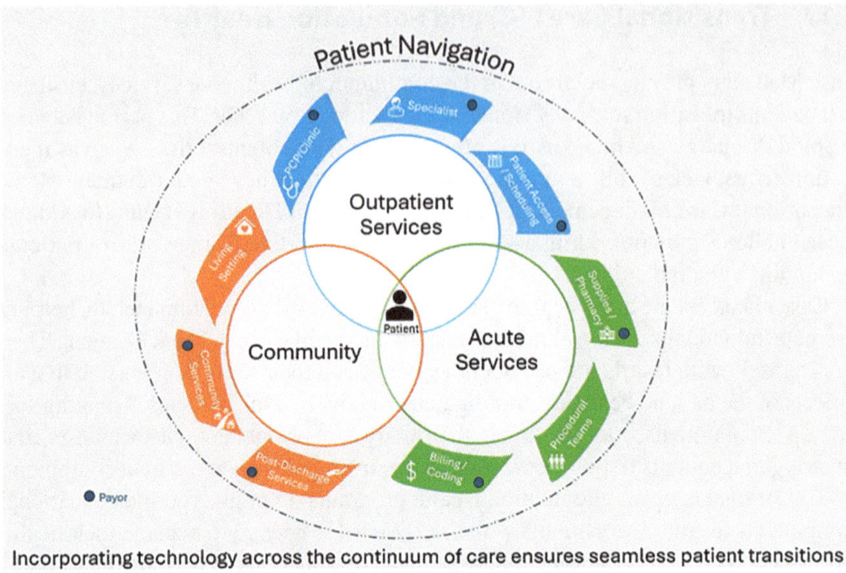

Fig. 5.5 Coordination care and information sharing across the continuum of care incorporating the patients payor benefits supports seamless transitions between care providers and eliminates inconsistencies. Created by the author

a sustainable healthcare system that prioritizes both quality outcomes and cost-efficiency (Fig. 5.5).

Investing in Transitional Care and Population Health is an investment in the future of healthcare. As the population ages and the prevalence of chronic conditions increases, the demand for seamless care transitions will only grow. By expanding and enhancing Transitional Care and Population Health programs, healthcare providers can meet this demand, ultimately fostering a healthier society where patients are supported throughout their recovery journey (Fig. 5.5).

5.18 Targeted Case Management (TCM)

Targeted Case Managers play a crucial role in supporting patients enrolled in state-managed Medicaid programs. These trained professionals are dedicated to assisting individuals who may be eligible for a range of additional services, which can be pivotal in promoting their health and well-being. One of the key components of this assistance is the role of Transitional Care Managers, who guide patients through the often complex processes involved in accessing necessary services.

The overarching goal of the Targeted Case Management program is to bridge gaps in care and significantly reduce hospital readmission rates among vulnerable populations. By providing tailored resources and support, these case managers help patients navigate their healthcare journeys, ensuring they receive comprehensive care that meets their unique needs.

Services offered under this program are diverse and aimed at enhancing the overall quality of life for patients. They encompass a variety of domains, including:

Medical and Clinical Care: Coordinating with healthcare providers to ensure that patients receive appropriate medical attention, follow-up appointments, and necessary treatments.

Social Services: Connecting patients with vital social services that may include housing assistance, transportation services, and community resources that provide support for day-to-day living.

Educational Services: Offering education about managing health conditions, understanding treatment options, and promoting healthy lifestyle choices that empower patients to take an active role in their health.

Given the diverse needs of the Medicaid population, it's essential for Targeted Case Managers to stay well-informed about the specific requirements and resources available within their state. Each state implements its own regulations, which may include unique training and certification processes for Case Managers. Therefore, it is imperative for professionals in this field to actively engage with state authorities and stay abreast of any changes in policies or programs.

The role of Targeted Case Managers extends beyond the immediate medical and social needs of the patients. They also work closely with family members and caregivers to ensure that the patient's support system is robust and well-coordinated. This holistic approach involves not only addressing the medical conditions of the patients but also considering their emotional and psychological well-being. Family members are often provided with resources and guidance on how to best support their loved ones during their recovery or ongoing care.

Targeted Case Managers are instrumental in advocating for their patients. They often work with legal entities and advocacy groups to ensure that the rights of the patients are upheld and that they receive the necessary support without any form of discrimination. This advocacy can include helping patients with disability claims, ensuring they have access to appropriate healthcare coverage, and navigating the complexities of government assistance programs.

Another critical aspect of Targeted Case Management is the focus on preventive care. Case Managers often coordinate preventive health screenings and educational workshops aimed at preventing the onset of chronic diseases. By proactively addressing potential health issues, case managers help reduce the long-term healthcare costs and improve the overall health outcomes of the population they serve.

Finally, the continuous professional development of Targeted Case Managers is essential for the success of the program. Regular training sessions, workshops, and conferences are conducted to ensure that these professionals are equipped with the latest knowledge and skills. This ongoing education allows them to stay updated with the evolving healthcare landscape and adopt best practices in their management strategies.

The work of Targeted Case Managers and Transitional Care Managers is vital in fostering optimal health outcomes for patients. By ensuring that individuals receive the appropriate support and resources, these professionals contribute to a more effective healthcare system, ultimately leading to healthier communities.

5.19 Community Liaison

Community liaison case managers hold a pivotal role in the healthcare industry, acting as essential liaisons between healthcare facilities, community providers, and the diverse populations they serve. Their multifaceted responsibilities make them a cornerstone of patient care, particularly in the realms of post-acute and community-based services. As the primary points of contact, case managers cultivate strong, positive relationships with community providers, which facilitates open lines of communication and collaboration. These connections are invaluable for patients, offering them a reliable resource with whom they can discuss their evolving needs and navigate the complexities of their healthcare journey.

In addition to fostering professional relationships with healthcare providers, case managers prioritize building trust and rapport with patients and their families. Through consistent and compassionate interactions, they create a safe space where patients can voice their concerns, ask questions, and engage in their own care process. This relationship not only empowers patients but also encourages them to trust the case manager's recommendations for additional resources, whether those be specialists, community services, or options related to their insurance or financial support.

The trust and understanding developed through these relationships are crucial, as they often lead to more efficient and effective healthcare delivery. Case managers can proactively identify potential barriers to care and address them before they escalate, resulting in a smoother transition between care providers and ultimately better health outcomes for patients.

Case managers play a crucial role in navigating the often-complicated landscape of healthcare services. They are equipped to advocate for patients, ensuring that their voices are heard and that they receive appropriate care tailored to their unique circumstances. By coordinating among various healthcare entities, hospitals, clinics, rehabilitation centers, and community organizations, case managers help streamline processes and eliminate redundancies, which can enhance the overall patient experience. They also provide crucial support during transitions between different levels of care, ensuring that patients do not feel overwhelmed or lost as they move from one provider to another. This continuity of care is essential in preventing gaps that could lead to setbacks or complications in a patient's health journey.

In addition, case managers often engage in continuous learning and professional development to stay abreast of the latest healthcare trends and best practices. This dedication to ongoing education allows them to offer the most current and effective solutions to the patients they serve. They might attend conferences, participate in workshops, or complete certifications that enhance their knowledge and skills, ultimately benefiting the patients who rely on their expertise.

Overall, the role of a case manager is critical not only in ensuring quality care but also in reinforcing the healthcare system's capacity to address the diverse needs of patients. Their expertise in bridging various entities within the healthcare landscape contributes significantly to achieving positive health outcomes, ensuring that each patient receives comprehensive, compassionate care tailored to their individual needs. Through their dedication and skill, case managers foster a more connected and effective healthcare delivery system, ultimately leading to healthier communities.

5.20 Case Manager as Educator

Case Managers play an indispensable role in the healthcare system by providing comprehensive educational support to patients, families, fellow healthcare providers, staff, and the broader community. Serving as patient advocates, Case Managers are adept at identifying individual patient needs and addressing them effectively. Their extensive training and knowledge empower them to educate patients about their health conditions, treatment options, available services, and additional resources that can facilitate their journey toward optimal health.

One of their critical responsibilities is to support patients and families during pivotal transitions in health, which can often be accompanied by challenging decisions. Case Managers offer not only emotional support but also practical resources, connecting patients with other healthcare providers and services tailored to their unique circumstances. This holistic approach helps to alleviate stress and ensures that patients feel informed and supported as they navigate the complexities of the healthcare system. Through regular consultations, Case Managers help patients understand the implications of their health conditions, treatment plans, and recovery processes. They provide detailed information and clarification on medical jargon that can often be confusing for patients and their families, ensuring that they are well-prepared to make informed decisions.

Beyond direct patient interactions, Case Managers also engage in the continuing education of other healthcare professionals. By sharing best practices for connecting patients with appropriate services, they enhance overall care delivery and improve health outcomes. This commitment to education ensures that all members of the healthcare team are equipped with the latest knowledge and strategies for effective patient management. Case Managers conduct workshops and seminars for healthcare staff, providing updates on new healthcare policies, treatment protocols, and patient care techniques. These educational sessions promote collaborative practice and help healthcare teams stay abreast of advancements in medical science and patient care technologies.

Case Managers take an active role in community outreach. They participate in health fairs, in-service training, and outreach initiatives at senior centers, assisted living facilities, and independent living communities. These efforts not only raise awareness about the role of Case Management but also empower patients to take an active role in their health. By fostering community connections, Case Managers help individuals understand how to effectively transition across various levels of care within the healthcare continuum. Additionally, they collaborate with local organizations to host informational sessions on preventative health measures, chronic disease management, and the importance of regular health screenings. These initiatives seek to improve community health literacy and encourage proactive health management among residents.

In their dedication to advancing the profession, Case Managers also assume the role of educators for future generations of nurses and social workers. By sharing their wealth of knowledge and experience within nursing programs, they provide budding professionals with a valuable foundation for patient care. This mentorship helps ensure that new nurses and social workers are well-prepared to deliver compassionate, informed care to their patients. Case Managers often serve as guest lecturers at universities and colleges, discussing real-world case studies and the evolving landscape of healthcare. Their insights and experiences provide students with a practical understanding of the challenges and rewards of Case Management.

Overall, Case Management is a vital specialty that significantly enhances the quality of healthcare delivered to patients. By combining the expertise of nursing and social work, Case Managers form a dynamic and efficient team devoted to improving patient outcomes and enriching the healthcare system as a whole. Their multifaceted role not only supports the patients they work with directly but also has a far-reaching impact on the entire community, making health education and advocacy accessible to all. Through their dedicated efforts, Case Managers contribute to a more informed, healthier society, where patients receive the comprehensive support they need to navigate their health journeys successfully.

5.21 Case Studies

Readmission Prevention

A 38-year-old patient returns to the Emergency Department (ED) 2 days after discharge from the hospital after completion of treatment for acute renal failure and pneumonia. The Case Manager met with the patient after identifying the ED readmission status while reviewing patient records.

During the assessment, the patient stated, "I was feeling great when I left here, but I don't feel good again." The Case Manager employed critical thinking and effective interview techniques. The patient shared that the medication was more expensive than expected, and they could not afford to fill it. Since all symptoms had been resolved, the medicine was no longer needed. The patient also stated that they were told to drink plenty of fluids and, since discharge, "I increased my fluid intake and have been drinking my coffee and diet soda." The Case Manager identified that the patient's health literacy potentially led to the current ED visit along with financial concerns.

The Case Manager discussed the assessment outcome with the ED provider, and a lower cost medication was identified. The Case Manager also located a medication discount card for that medicine online.

The nurse and Case Manager provided education to the patient regarding the type and amount of fluid that should be added to the patient's daily routine. This included drinking at least 1 glass of water every hour, with an example glass shown to the patient for size reference. The patient was able to repeat the education, demonstrating an understanding of their health care needs.

Did the Case Manager prevent an unnecessary hospital readmission?

The patient was successfully discharged from the ED with an affordable medication that was called into the pharmacy for pickup with the discount applied. The patient was also notified of the cost during the discharge process. The patient also received discharge information tailored to their health literacy level.

Multidisciplinary Rounds and Complex Case

During daily Multidisciplinary Rounds, a 71-year-old patient was presented and discussed. The patient is on day 2 of admission for Congestive Heart Failure (CHF) exacerbation with a complex history of poorly controlled Chronic Obstructive Pulmonary Disease (COPD), Chronic Kidney Disease (CKD) stage 3, and poorly controlled Diabetes (DM).

Therapy states that the patient is too weak to get out of bed, and due to the use of the monitors, safety was a concern. They have been encouraging the patient to change positions in bed and to sit in bed as tolerated. Nursing reports that the patient's urinary output has decreased, and shortness of breath is continuing; the patient is receiving 5 liters of oxygen via nasal canula. Lab values remain elevated. A nutritionist states that education is being provided to the patient and family regarding a low-sodium diet to reduce the risk of fluid retention. The case management assessment information included the patient living alone in a "mother suite" in the family's backyard and having been independent prior to discharge, except for driving, which the family manages as needed. The provider discussed the balance required to allow for diuresis at a slow rate to avoid a potential negative impact on renal function. The expected discharge date is unknown at present.

Based on this information, what would the Case Manager want to evaluate or discuss?

The Case Manager would want to coordinate with therapy, provider, patient, and family to determine discharge needs, which may include post-acute services, and initiate referrals to multiple levels of care for initial evaluations and monitoring of the condition to determine the final discharge plan and avoid potential delays in transition to the next appropriate level.

The Utilization Review team should also be made aware of this discussion for inclusion in communication with the payor.

If the facility has Complex Case Rounds, this case would be appropriate for escalation to receive additional clinical discussion, monitoring, and potential recommendations for the care plan.

Reporting and Monitoring

6

Learning Objectives

1. **Understand Compliance Framework:** Explain the importance of compliance within the healthcare system, particularly in relation to regulatory requirements established by the Centers for Medicare and Medicaid Services (CMS).
2. **Reporting and Monitoring Processes:** Discuss the processes involved in reporting and monitoring compliance, patient outcomes and care provision are impacted by Case Management teams.
3. **Impact on Patient Outcomes:** Assess the effectiveness of monitoring and reporting key data in achieving improved health outcomes for patients and enhanced operational integrity for healthcare organizations.
4. **Data-Driven Decision Making:** Analyze how data analytics can be employed to identify areas of opportunity to improve patient care, patient outcomes, and facility revenue.

6.1 Compliance

Compliance is an essential aspect of the healthcare system, with Case Management playing a pivotal role in ensuring that various dimensions of patient care meet the highest standards of quality and compliance. This specifically pertains to regulatory requirements established by the Centers for Medicare and Medicaid Services (CMS). Case Management responsibilities are not only fundamental to patient care but also integral to the operational integrity of healthcare organizations that participate in

S. Garceau, *Interdisciplinary Case Management: A Nursing Practice Approach*,
https://doi.org/10.1007/978-3-032-20960-3_6

Medicare and Medicaid programs. As the healthcare landscape evolves, the importance of continuous compliance with these regulations becomes increasingly critical.

Central to the Case Management function is the recognition and advocacy of patient's rights, which are paramount in fostering a supportive healthcare environment. Case Managers are entrusted with upholding and promoting essential rights, including:

- The right to receive competent and appropriate care that meets their unique health needs.
- The right to provide informed consent or refuse treatment based on comprehensive understanding.
- The right to access emergency medical care, irrespective of payment capabilities or insurance network affiliations.
- The right to confidentiality surrounding their personal health information, ensuring privacy and trust.
- The right to continuity of care, which requires facilitating smooth transitions through various levels of care and services, thereby minimizing disruptions in treatment.

In this sensitive arena of healthcare, Case Managers serve as essential advocates, guiding patients and their families through complex medical decisions and processes. This role becomes particularly critical when patients encounter challenges related to their medical conditions, age, or comorbidities that may impede their ability to make informed choices. Ethical principles, such as respect for patient autonomy and beneficence, must continually be at the forefront of Case Managers' actions, especially when facilitating the involvement of designated decision-makers in care discussions and fostering collaborative decision-making processes that prioritize patient well-being.

Compliance with CMS requirements constitutes a significant aspect of Case Management, specifically through the Conditions of Participation that healthcare organizations must satisfy to maintain access to Medicare and Medicaid funding. A vital component of this compliance is the engagement of Case Management in the Utilization Review process, often led by the Utilization Review Committee. Case Managers play a critical role in gathering, compiling, and presenting necessary information to this committee, supporting decisions that align with CMS guidelines while consistently emphasizing the importance of patient-centered care.

Discharge planning is yet another crucial responsibility of Case Management. Upon discharge, patients retain the autonomy to select their preferred healthcare providers, and it is the duty of healthcare facilities to adhere to stringent regulations, such as the Stark Law. This law is particularly designed to prevent conflicts of interest by prohibiting healthcare providers from making referrals to entities in which they have financial relationships. Ensuring adherence to this law is essential for maintaining ethical standards and safeguarding patients' best interests.

In the hospital environment, patients receive written documentation detailing their rights. This is a fundamental aspect of comprehensive care that aligns with the Utilization Review process. This documentation assists in determining the appropriate level of care status—whether Inpatient or Observation—based on clinical documentation and physician judgment. Patients and their representatives possess the right to contest any decisions made regarding their level of care or discharge orders, especially if they feel that the timing is premature. Important documents, particularly the Important Message from Medicare, the Medicare Outpatient Observation Notice, and the Hospital Notice of Noncoverage, are standard tools utilized to effectively communicate these rights. Currently, four main forms are systematically used for these communications: HINN 1, HINN 10, HINN 11, and HINN 12.

To maintain compliance and address any issues that may arise, all layers of compliance are reported systematically to the Board of Directors, either via the Utilization Review Committee or the Utilization Management Committee. It is imperative for healthcare organizations to diligently track compliance and tackle any concerns promptly, as their ability to participate in Medicare and Medicaid programs is closely tied to adherence to federal regulations. Ensuring compliance not only secures essential funding but also reinforces the organization's unwavering commitment to delivering high-quality, ethical healthcare to all patients, thereby enhancing overall health outcomes and fostering a culture of accountability and excellence within the healthcare system.

6.2 Key Performance Indicators

Healthcare providers and facilities rely on Key Performance Indicators (KPI) as essential tools for monitoring and enhancing various aspects of patient care. By establishing specific KPI, organizations can create a structured framework that not only highlights areas needing improvement but also fosters a culture of accountability and excellence in patient services. These indicators serve as a compass, guiding organizations toward their goals and ensuring that patient care remains at the forefront of their mission.

Different healthcare providers implement a diverse range of data collection tools and methodologies to assess performance. Common tools include Electronic Medical Records (EMRs), spreadsheets, and visual dashboards designed to synthesize complex data into actionable insights. Despite the variety of tools available, it is crucial to emphasize that consistency in tracking key performance areas is more significant than the specific tools employed. This continuity ensures that potential deficits can be identified effectively, and necessary improvements can be systematically applied to enhance overall patient care and operational efficiency.

KPI are not static; they evolve as strategic priorities shift within the organization or as external healthcare environments change. For instance, Case Management KPI often focus on critical metrics such as patient census and length of stay for both inpatient and observation cases. Monitoring variances between the actual length of stay (ALOS) and the Diagnosis-Related Group (DRG) geometric length of stay (GLOS or GMLOS) is vital for identifying operational efficiencies and opportunities for reduced costs. Another important aspect is the analysis of data related to short-stay and extended-stay cases, as well as compliance with the Centers for Medicare & Medicaid Services (CMS) notice distribution. The timing of discharge assessments must also be closely monitored to ensure best practices are consistently followed across the board.

In addition, other pertinent KPI may include the involvement of a Physician Advisor, along with data supporting their role, which can play a significant role in improving patient outcomes. Metrics related to avoidable days and delays, readmission rates, denial statistics, and discharge data must be included as well. By incorporating these diverse KPI, healthcare organizations can construct a comprehensive view of performance that identifies both strengths and areas for growth, allowing for a more nuanced understanding of operational realities.

The systematic collection and monitoring of KPI is essential for recognizing when performance deviates from established benchmarks. This proactive approach allows healthcare providers to develop targeted strategies that enhance patient care, address identified gaps, and optimize resource allocation. KPI reports serve as a vital component in illustrating the value of Case Management programs to executive leadership. Data-driven insights into patient outcomes, combined with business operational efficiencies, equip decision-makers with the compelling evidence needed to evaluate and endorse the significance of Case Management roles within the facility.

Leveraging KPIs effectively not only informs healthcare practitioners about their operational performance but also supports strategic initiatives aimed at improving patient outcomes and overall facility efficiency. Establishing a robust framework for KPI utilization is integral to continuous quality improvement in healthcare settings. By rigorously measuring performance and identifying areas for enhancement, organizations can take proactive steps toward achieving better patient experiences. Ultimately, this leads to enhanced organizational success, ensuring that healthcare systems remain resilient and capable of providing high-quality care to the communities they serve.

6.3 Physician Advisor Engagement

The Physician Advisor is engaged to support both Case Management and Utilization Management by providing clinical expertise and guidance on complex cases, facilitating communication between physicians and case managers, and ensuring adherence to regulatory requirements and best practice standards. Their involvement is crucial in resolving disputes regarding patient status, clarifying medical necessity, and assisting with denial management processes. By serving as a liaison and resource, the Physician Advisor helps optimize care delivery, improve documentation, and enhance overall patient outcomes within the healthcare organization.

The Physician Advisor is also available to assist attending providers with additional medical expertise to overcome plateaus in patient recovery and support patient throughput that is aligned with the patient's medical progress.

6.4 Case Management Value Reflected in Data

By tracking, trending, and reporting objective data using Key Performance Indicators, the Case Management team will be able to demonstrate the impact on regulation compliance, patient throughput, patient satisfaction, readmission rates, and facility revenue. Following leading practice standards of work will support improvement in these strategic areas. Leadership will be able to relate the valuable work performed by all areas of Case Management which will lend further administrative support to evolve the practice to meet additional patient population needs.

Case Management as a Profession

7

Learning Objectives

1. **Career Advancement Opportunities:** Recognize the potential for professional growth within the field of Case Management and explore pathways to elevate one's nursing career through specialization.
2. **Curriculum Components:** Learn about the key areas covered in Case Management or Care Coordination master's degree programs, including clinical practices, healthcare policy, financial management, and ethical decision-making.
3. **Skills Development:** Identify the advanced skills and knowledge necessary to effectively address the complexities of patient care and improve overall health outcomes.
4. **The Importance of Education:** Understand how pursuing further education in Case Management can enhance career prospects and equip professionals to meet the evolving needs of patient populations.

The time has come to elevate your nursing career to exciting new heights. The healthcare industry is evolving rapidly, and there has never been a more promising moment to specialize in Case Management. This growing field emphasizes a fundamental shift towards comprehensive and effective care for patients, which is essential in an increasingly complex healthcare environment. With an increasing number of colleges and universities offering Case Management or Care Coordination as specialized master's degree programs, you have a unique opportunity to enrich both your education and your career prospects.

Pursuing a master's degree in Case Management equips you with advanced knowledge and skills that are highly sought after in today's healthcare landscape. These programs not

S. Garceau, *Interdisciplinary Case Management: A Nursing Practice Approach*,
https://doi.org/10.1007/978-3-032-20960-3_7

only cover clinical aspects but also delve into areas such as healthcare policy, financial management, and ethical decision-making. This comprehensive education prepares you to tackle the multifaceted challenges that arise in patient care and ensures that you are prepared to manage diverse cases effectively. Additionally, obtaining specialty certifications in various subspecialties of Case Management can significantly enhance your employability and professional credibility. These certifications demonstrate your commitment to the field and can set you apart in a competitive job market.

Being recognized as a well-trained and educated Case Management professional not only positions you as a valuable asset to healthcare organizations but also empowers you to influence and improve healthcare programs. You become an integral part of a team dedicated to ensuring that patients receive the most appropriate and efficient care. By coordinating between various stakeholders including patients, families, healthcare providers, insurance companies, you can help facilitate clearer communication and ultimately improve patient outcomes.

National associations play a pivotal role in supporting Case Management professionals. Organizations such as the American Case Management Association (ACMA), National Association of Case Management (NACM), Case Management Society of America (CMSA), Commission for Case Manager Certification (CCMC), and Health Utilization Management Accreditation (URAC) are committed to the advancement of Case Management. These associations provide valuable resources, networking opportunities, and professional development. Joining such organizations allows you to connect with other professionals in the field, share insights, and access a wealth of information that can enhance your practice. These professional organizations often host conferences, webinars, and workshops that facilitate continuous learning, keeping you up to date with industry standards and best practices.

As the scope of Case Management continues to expand, there is a burgeoning demand for expertise in areas such as Utilization Review, Care Coordination, Targeted Case Management, Transitional Care Management, and Denial Management. These areas are critical not only for improving patient outcomes but also for enhancing the operational efficacy of healthcare systems. The significance of these services is increasingly being recognized by healthcare executives who understand their critical impact on patient outcomes and operational efficiency. For instance, robust Case Management programs have been proven to enhance patient experiences, improve satisfaction rates, and help healthcare providers function more effectively and efficiently. This positive impact extends beyond individual patients to entire communities, bolstering public health initiatives and reducing healthcare costs for organizations and patients alike.

The notion that "a nurse is a nurse" is becoming obsolete. Healthcare providers are now appreciating the immense value that comes from specialized knowledge and skills. As such, embracing the role of a Case Management specialist positions you at the forefront of this transformation within the healthcare industry. This shift is paramount as healthcare systems face increased scrutiny regarding their effectiveness and efficiency, making the role of Case Managers even more vital in navigating these challenges.

By committing to ongoing education and expertise development, you can elevate your career trajectory while significantly contributing to improved healthcare outcomes for patients and communities. Consider the diverse opportunities available to you; whether working in hospitals, outpatient settings, or even within insurance companies, the possibilities are vast. Each setting presents unique challenges and learning experiences that can shape your career and allow you to make meaningful contributions to the healthcare system.

In addition to clinical roles, Case Management can open doors to leadership positions in healthcare organizations. Specialists in this field are often sought after for their ability to navigate complex cases, advocate for patients, and implement strategies that improve interdisciplinary collaboration. As you grow in your career, consider pursuing administrative roles where you can influence organizational policies and contribute to the future direction of healthcare delivery.

Engaging with patients is at the heart of Case Management. You're not just managing cases; you are advocating for individuals navigating a complex system, ensuring they receive the necessary resources, education, and support. It's about understanding their unique circumstances—medical, social, and emotional—and tailoring interventions that best meet their needs. The relationships you build with patients can be life-changing, not only for them but for you as well. There's immense satisfaction in seeing a patient achieve their health goals, knowing you played a part in that journey.

Now is the time to take that first bold step toward becoming a Case Management specialist. Invest in your future, enhance your skill set, and play a vital role in shaping the future of healthcare. The journey toward specialization begins today! Consider looking at various programs and certifications that align with your career goals and interests. Research different educational institutions and the types of courses they offer, whether in-person or online, to find the best fit for your needs.

Additionally, explore the possibility of internships or mentorships in the field of Case Management. These experiences can provide invaluable hands-on knowledge and insights that will further prepare you for your future career. Establishing connections with experienced professionals can guide you through your educational journey and help you navigate early career decisions.

Don't underestimate the power of networking. Attend local chapter meetings of professional organizations and connect with peers who share your passion for Case Management. These relationships can offer support, resources, and referrals that benefit your career in ways you might not yet imagine. Engage with social media platforms, such as LinkedIn, where you can join groups and discussions dedicated to Case Management topics. This engagement can keep you informed on industry trends and enrich your understanding of the challenges and innovations within the field.

Specializing in Case Management represents a significant opportunity for personal and professional growth. It allows you to transcend traditional nursing roles and become a leader in a rapidly evolving healthcare landscape. By prioritizing your education and embracing the responsibilities of a Case Management specialist, you will play a crucial role in improving healthcare delivery and outcomes for diverse populations. Step forward on this path with confidence, and remember that the impact you make today can shape the healthcare systems of tomorrow. The future is bright, and the role of Case Management is set to become even more integral to how healthcare is provided in the years to come.

Looking to the Future

8

Learning Objectives

1. **Understand the Evolution of Case Management:** Describe the historical context and changes within the Case Management specialty in nursing, focusing on technological advancements and healthcare policy shifts.
2. **Apply Technology in Case Management:** Analyze the role of technology, including electronic health records (EHRs) and AI-driven analytics, in improving communication, monitoring patient progress, and enhancing decision-making.
3. **Critically Reflect on Future Trends in Case Management:** Explore emerging trends and innovations within the Case Management field, considering how they can lead to improved care delivery models and overall health outcomes.

The nursing field is in a state of perpetual evolution, influenced by scientific advancements, shifts in patient needs, and the ever-changing landscape of healthcare policy. Among the many specialties that are adapting to these shifts, Case Management stands out as the fastest-growing nursing specialty. With the integration of technological innovations and advancements in medical science, healthcare delivery is undergoing significant transformation. In this dynamic environment, the role of healthcare professionals has become increasingly crucial in helping patients attain optimal health outcomes. This journey encompasses not only the recovery from illnesses and injuries but also effective management of chronic diseases and the complexities that accompany aging.

Case Management plays a pivotal role in this transformative journey. It offers structured support and guidance for both patients and healthcare providers, thereby

S. Garceau, *Interdisciplinary Case Management: A Nursing Practice Approach*,
https://doi.org/10.1007/978-3-032-20960-3_8

facilitating a patient-centric approach to care. By establishing partnerships between patients and various healthcare professionals, Case Management becomes instrumental in identifying innovative, tailored approaches to care. This collaboration aims to empower patients along their health journeys, ensuring comprehensive support at every stage of their lives.

The practice of Case Management also calls for a multi-faceted understanding of healthcare delivery systems, including the roles that social determinants of health play in patient outcomes. With growing recognition of the significant impact that socio-economic factors have on health, Case Managers must advocate not only for individual patients but also for broader systemic changes that address these inequalities. Training future generations of Case Management professionals necessitates a robust foundation of knowledge about the current state of the profession, alongside an awareness of external factors that may impact care delivery.

As we look towards the future of healthcare, one thing is clear: Case Management will continue to be an integral component of patient advocacy and health improvement. Healthcare systems increasingly recognize the value of Case Management in leading the charge toward innovative care delivery models, which not only benefit individual patients but also enhance health outcomes for populations at large. The journey of growing the Case Management specialty is one of compassion, continuous improvement, and learning, aimed at ensuring that each patient continues to receive the personalized support they require in a rapidly changing healthcare environment.

8.1 Artificial Intelligence (AI) and Automation in Case Management

The future of Case Management is not just on the horizon; it's unfolding right before our eyes, presenting an exhilarating time for healthcare professionals dedicated to this vital field. Traditional Case Management roles often centered around utilization reviews that assess the necessity and efficiency of medical services. This aspect has been crucial in ensuring that healthcare resources are allocated wisely and that patients receive the appropriate care they need. However, we are currently witnessing a transformative shift towards a more holistic, patient-centered approach that underscores the importance of care coordination and proactive patient follow-up.

Care coordination represents a multidisciplinary strategy where diverse healthcare providers work together seamlessly to ensure each patient's journey is not only smooth but effective. This integration is particularly vital for individuals with complex health needs, as it helps to eliminate communication gaps that can result in fragmented care, thereby minimizing the risk of medical errors. For healthcare providers, this offers the opportunity to pool collective expertise, fostering an environment where information sharing leads to better decision-making and care strategies.

Similarly, patient follow-up is emerging as a cornerstone of successful Case Management. By actively engaging patients after their initial treatment, healthcare providers can monitor progress and address any concerns that may arise, offering ongoing support throughout the recovery or management process. This continuous interaction fosters a strong rapport between patients and providers, encouraging individuals to take charge of their health journeys in ways that empower them. Maintaining this ongoing relationship not only enhances patient satisfaction but also increases adherence to treatment plans, which are critical for achieving desired health outcomes.

The role of technology and data analytics in these developments cannot be overstated. Innovative tools and platforms are emerging that enable case managers to track patient information with greater efficacy, enhancing communication channels and informed decision-making. For instance, electronic health records (EHRs) and telehealth platforms facilitate timely access to patient information and promote effective communication among care teams. The utilization of AI-driven analytics helps identify trends and patterns in patient behavior, allowing case managers to engage with patients more effectively and preemptively address potential issues before they escalate into crises.

The introduction of AI in Case Management also holds the promise of streamlining administrative processes and reducing the burden of paperwork. Automated systems can assist with scheduling appointments, sending reminders, and even documenting care, enabling case managers to focus their time and expertise on direct patient interaction and personalized care. This advancement not only enhances the overall efficiency of healthcare systems but also allows for a more human-centric approach where patient interactions become the focal point of care.

It is truly inspiring to witness how these changes are shaping the landscape of Case Management. As healthcare systems adapt to these new ideologies, we can expect to see increased collaboration, enriched patient experiences, and ultimately, superior health outcomes. This ongoing evolution reflects a growing recognition of the necessity for comprehensive care that addresses not just immediate medical issues but also a patient's overall well-being and quality of life.

For Case Management professionals, the future holds opportunities for specialization and advanced training. As the field grows, there will be a demand for case managers who are equipped to handle complex cases that integrate behavioral health, chronic disease management, and technological tools. Lifelong learning will be critical, as practitioners must stay current with health trends, policy changes, and advancements in technology that affect care coordination.

As we embark on this exciting journey, it's essential to remain focused on the core mission of Case Management: to provide compassionate, patient-centered care that optimally supports individuals' health while also aptly utilizing resources within healthcare systems. The future looks bright, and the commitment to embracing these transformative changes is vital. By continuously evolving and adapting to the intricacies of patient care, healthcare professionals can look forward to a landscape where innovation drives successful outcomes, delivering not only efficiency but also empathy and understanding in care. Through collaboration, advanced training, and the intelligent use of technology, Case Management can truly forge a path towards a future that prioritizes the health and welfare of patients, ensuring they receive the tailored support they deserve in a rapidly changing healthcare environment.

9 Workflows

Learning Objectives

1. **Utilize Structured Methodologies:** Explain how structured methodologies can enhance the effectiveness of case management by streamlining processes and improving health outcomes.
2. **Identify Learning Preferences:** Recognize different learning styles among practitioners and the importance of offering a variety of educational tools, such as instruction manuals and visual aids.
3. **Interpret Visual Workflows:** Demonstrate the ability to read and utilize visual workflows, such as decision trees and flowcharts, to navigate the case management process effectively.
4. **Implement Algorithms in Practice:** Apply algorithms and structured decision-making pathways in clinical scenarios to enhance patient care planning and execution.
5. **Evaluate Patient Needs Systematically:** Analyze patient cases using visual tools to identify critical decision points and ensure comprehensive assessment and intervention.

To effectively navigate the diverse functions and tasks associated with Case Management, it is beneficial to employ algorithms that parallel those utilized in other nursing procedures. Case Management involves coordinating patient care, resources, assessment, and follow-up to ensure optimal health outcomes. Given its complexity, implementing structured methodologies can streamline this process and enhance its effectiveness.

While some individuals may find it more effective to consult instruction manuals for guidance, others may prefer the clarity offered by visual aids, such as decision trees.

S. Garceau, *Interdisciplinary Case Management: A Nursing Practice Approach*,
https://doi.org/10.1007/978-3-032-20960-3_9

Each practitioner has unique learning styles and preferences, which is why providing a variety of tools is essential. Instruction manuals can offer detailed explanations and theoretical background, allowing nurses to understand the rationale behind each step. On the other hand, visual aids like flowcharts and diagrams can simplify complex information, making it more accessible.

This section is dedicated to presenting visual workflows that illustrate the case management process, allowing practitioners to easily reference and follow structured decision-making paths. These visual tools aim to enhance understanding by transforming verbose guidelines into intuitive visuals that map out each step in the patient care continuum. For example, a decision tree can outline potential patient scenarios and guide the practitioner through the options available for assessment, intervention, and evaluation.

Integrating algorithms and workflows into daily practice not only streamlines the process but also facilitates better patient outcomes. Visual tools can help practitioners quickly identify critical decision points, ensuring that no essential steps are overlooked. This approach fosters a thorough and systematic evaluation of patient needs and encourages proactive intervention, which is vital for managing complex cases effectively.

Additionally, training nursing professionals to utilize these algorithms can lead to a more cohesive approach to case management within healthcare teams. Collaboration and communication become more streamlined when all team members are using a common framework. This alignment can reduce misunderstandings, enhance teamwork, and promote a culture of continuous improvement in patient care.

By integrating these algorithms and workflows into their practice, nursing professionals can improve their case management strategies, leading to higher quality care and more effective resolution of complex patient needs. Ultimately, when case management is approached with structured methodologies and visual tools, it empowers healthcare providers to deliver informed, efficient, and empathetic care that directly impacts patient satisfaction and outcomes. Emphasizing these practices cultivates a nursing environment that is adaptable, knowledgeable, and prepared to meet the dynamic challenges of patient care.

The following workflows are foundational examples used successfully and may be modified to meet a specific facility's needs.

9.1 UM, CM, CDI Communication

See Fig. 9.1.

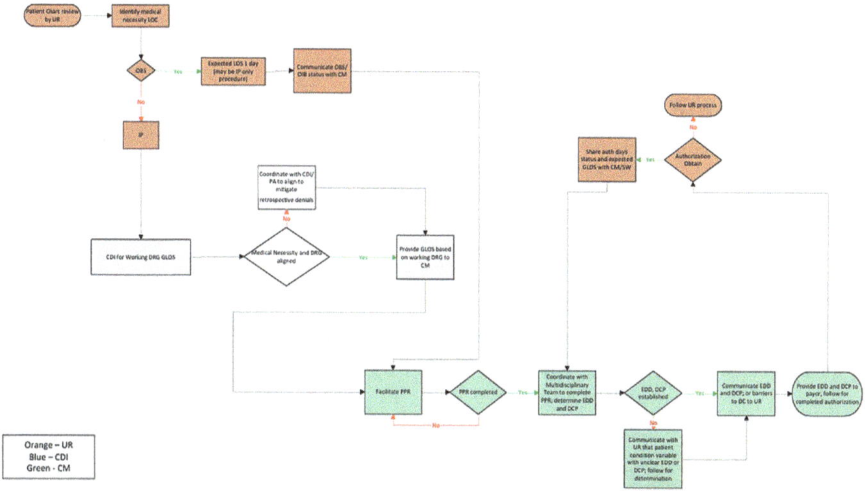

Fig. 9.1 A decision tree from the start of the process through the end as denoted by the oval shapes. Each diamond shape is a decision to be made following a yes or no pathway. Created by the author

9.2 Utilization Management Process Workflows

Many workflow processes apply specifically to the Utilization Management work and the coordination between all teams included in the Revenue Cycle. It is important that UM and CM work closely together as much of the work is communicated in a two-way process for successful and compliant completion.

High-Level Utilization Management Function

See Fig. 9.2.

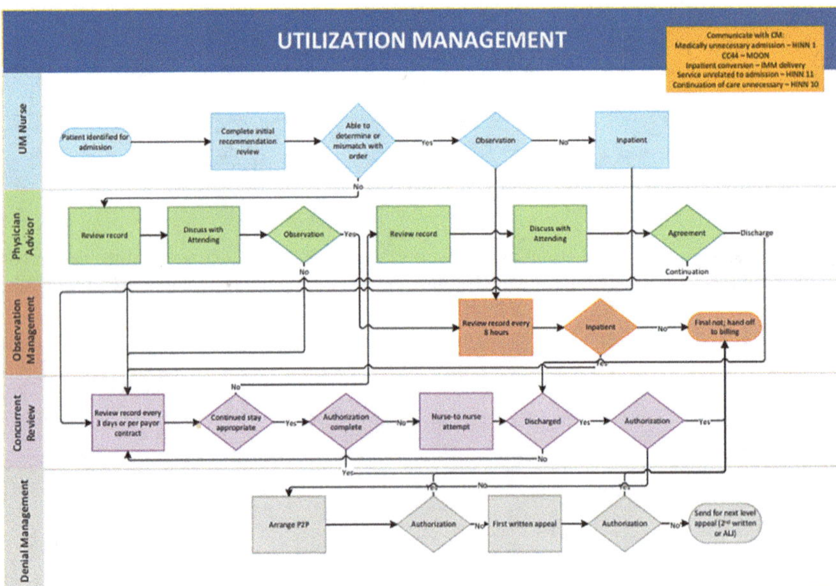

Fig. 9.2 A decision tree from the start of the process through the end as denoted by the oval shapes. Each diamond shape is a decision to be made following a yes or no pathway. Created by the author

Initial Review

See Fig. 9.3.

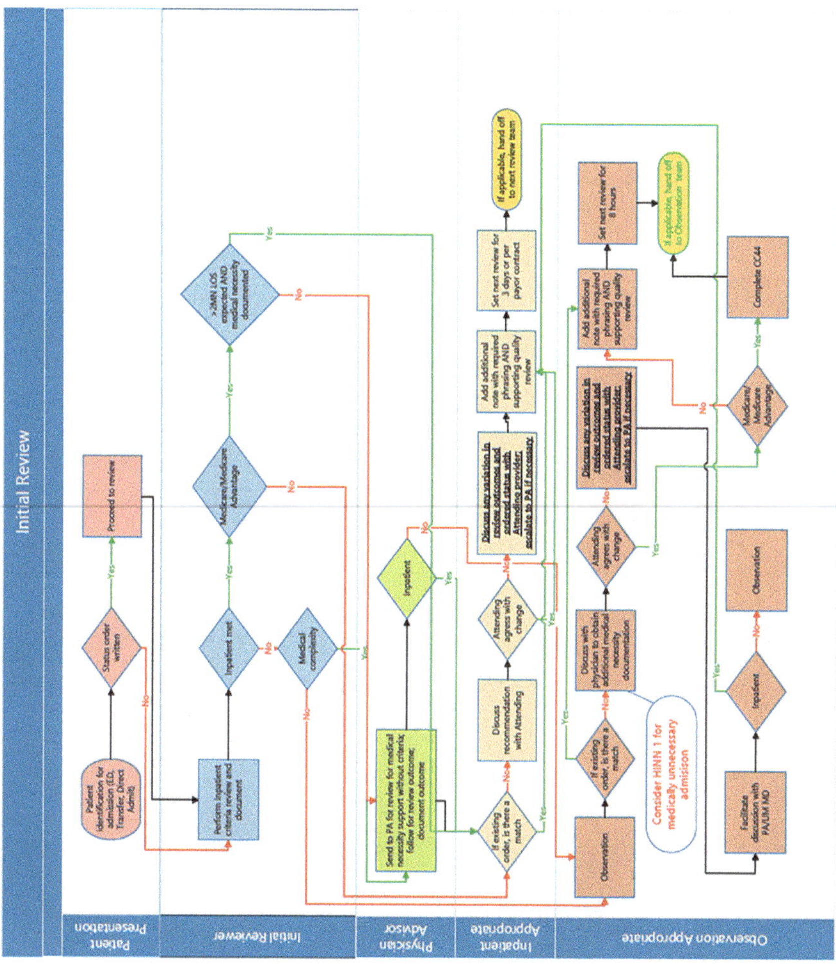

Fig. 9.3 A decision tree from the start of the process through the end as denoted by the oval shapes. Each diamond shape is a decision to be made following a yes or no pathway. Created by the author

Initial Review from the Logistic (Transfer) Center or Direct Admit

See Fig. 9.4.

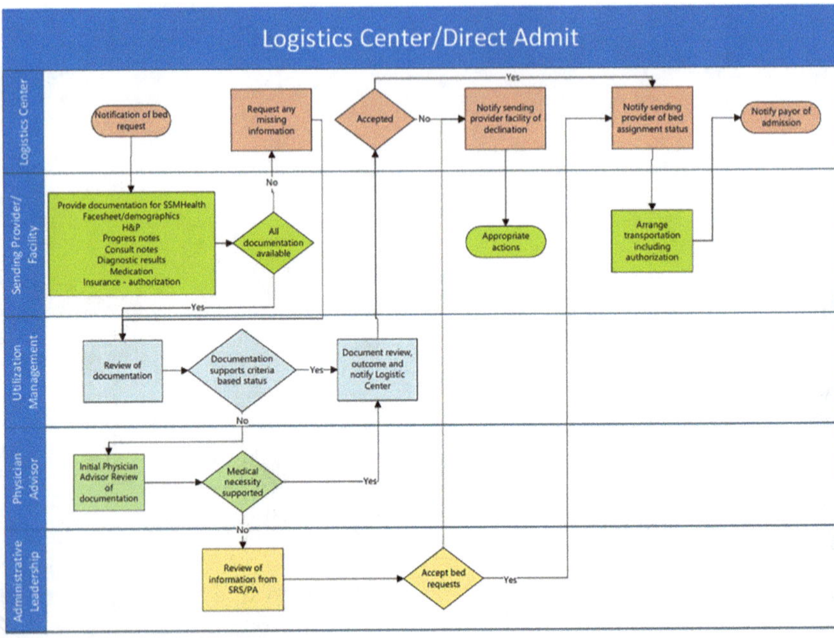

Fig. 9.4 A decision tree from the start of the process through the end as denoted by the oval shapes. Each diamond shape is a decision to be made following a yes or no pathway. Created by the author

Pre-Procedural

See Fig. 9.5.

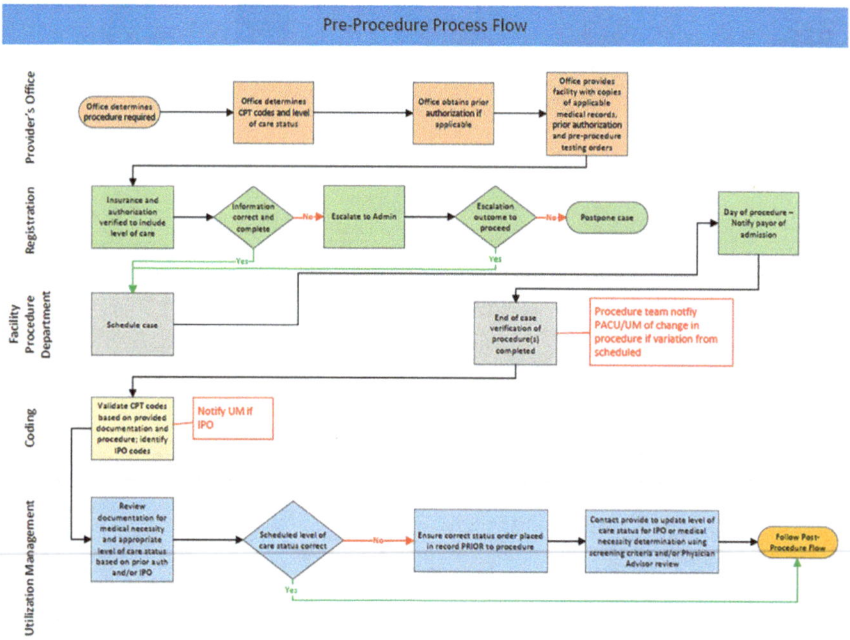

Fig. 9.5 A decision tree from the start of the process through the end as denoted by the oval shapes. Each diamond shape is a decision to be made following a yes or no pathway. Created by the author

Pre-Procedure Review and Discharge Assessment

Fig. 9.6

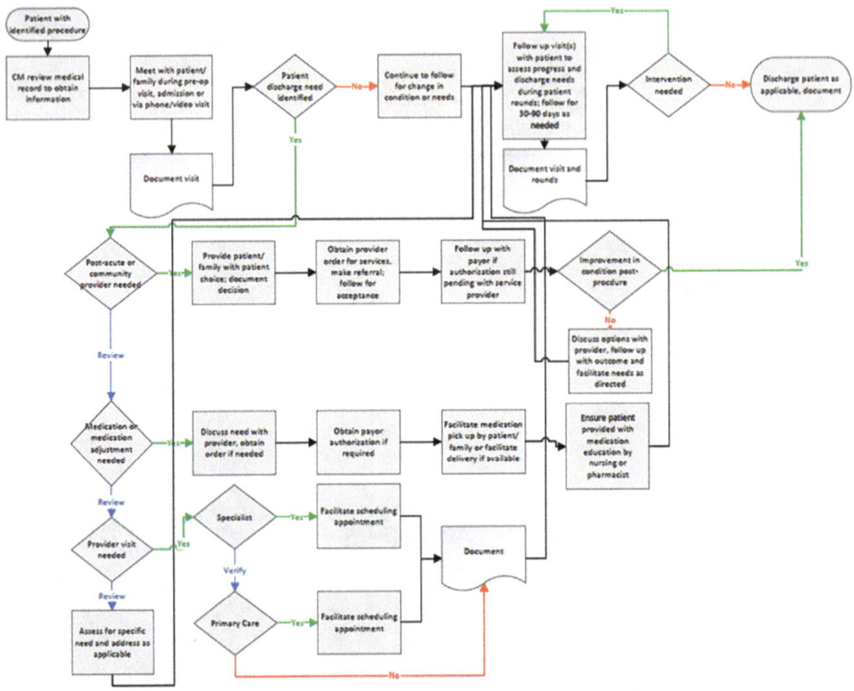

Fig. 9.6 A decision tree from the start of the process through the end as denoted by the oval shapes. Each diamond shape is a decision to be made following a yes or no pathway. Created by the author

Post-Procedure

See Fig. 9.7.

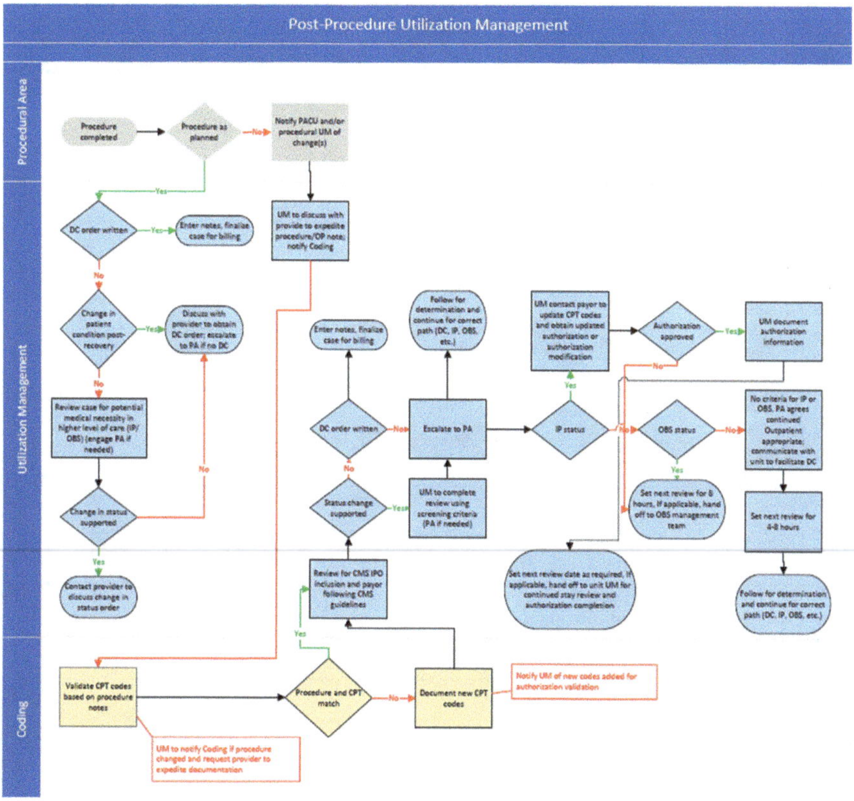

Fig. 9.7 A decision tree from the start of the process through the end as denoted by the oval shapes. Each diamond shape is a decision to be made following a yes or no pathway. Created by the author

Observation/Outpatient in a Bed Management

See Fig. 9.8.

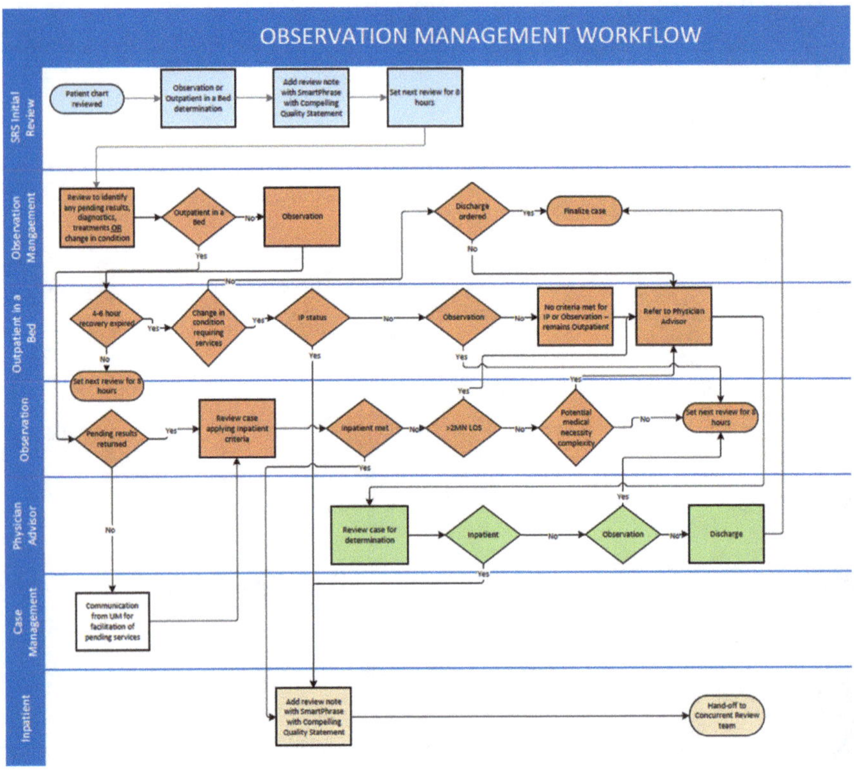

Fig. 9.8 A decision tree from the start of the process through the end as denoted by the oval shapes. Each diamond shape is a decision to be made following a yes or no pathway. Created by the author

MOON Process

See Fig. 9.9.

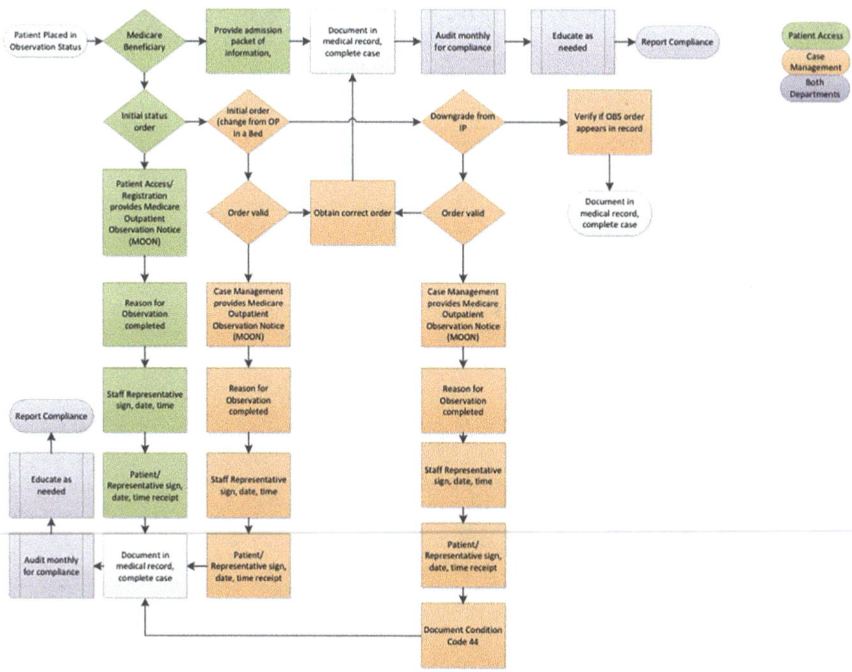

Fig. 9.9 A decision tree from the start of the process through the end as denoted by the oval shapes. Each diamond shape is a decision to be made following a yes or no pathway. Created by the author

Condition Code 44

See Fig. 9.10.

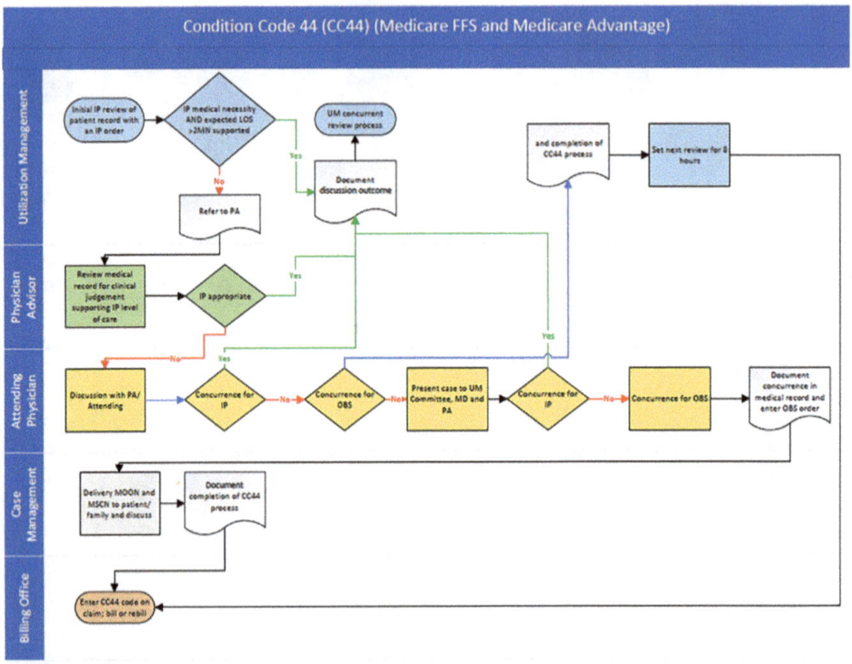

Fig. 9.10 A decision tree from the start of the process through the end as denoted by the oval shapes. Each diamond shape is a decision to be made following a yes or no pathway. Created by the author

Concurrent Review

See Fig. 9.11.

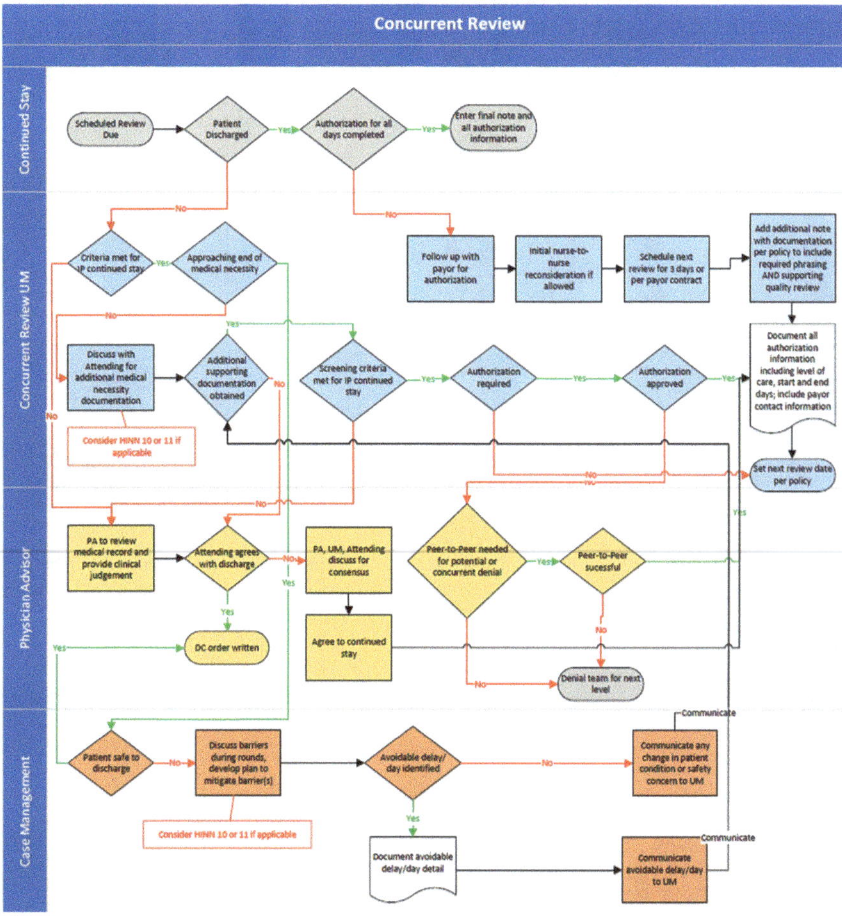

Fig. 9.11 A decision tree from the start of the process through the end as denoted by the oval shapes. Each diamond shape is a decision to be made following a yes or no pathway. Created by the author

Short-Stay Review

See Fig. 9.12.

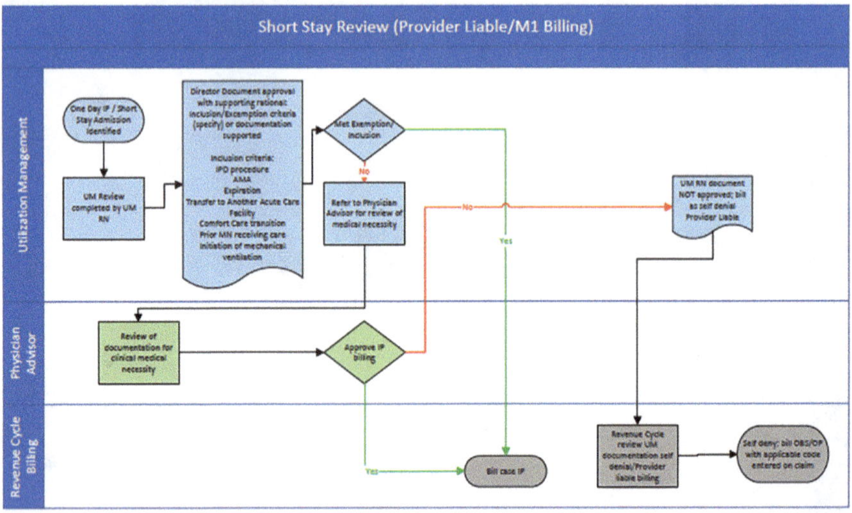

Fig. 9.12 A decision tree from the start of the process through the end as denoted by the oval shapes. Each diamond shape is a decision to be made following a yes or no pathway. Created by the author

Occurrence Span Code 72

See Fig. 9.13.

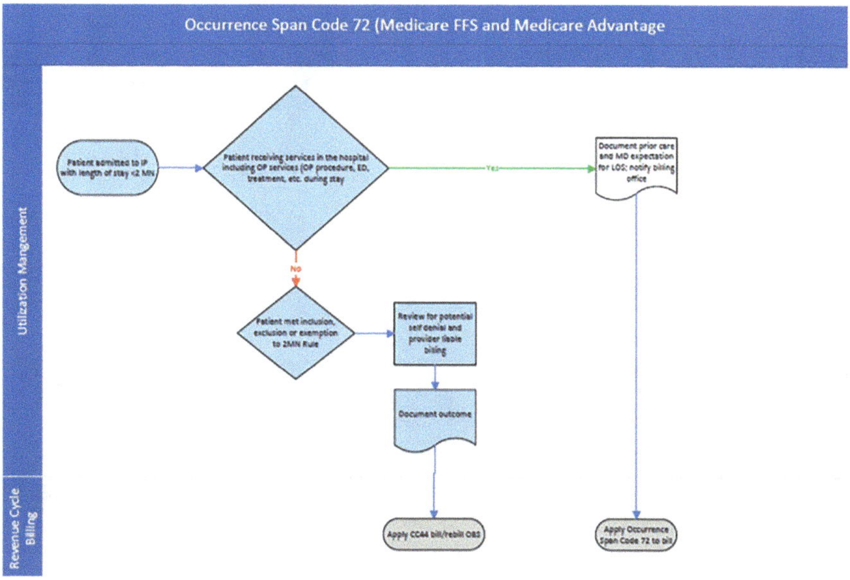

Fig. 9.13 A decision tree from the start of the process through the end as denoted by the oval shapes. Each diamond shape is a decision to be made following a yes or no pathway. Created by the author

Commercial Downgrade

See Fig. 9.14.

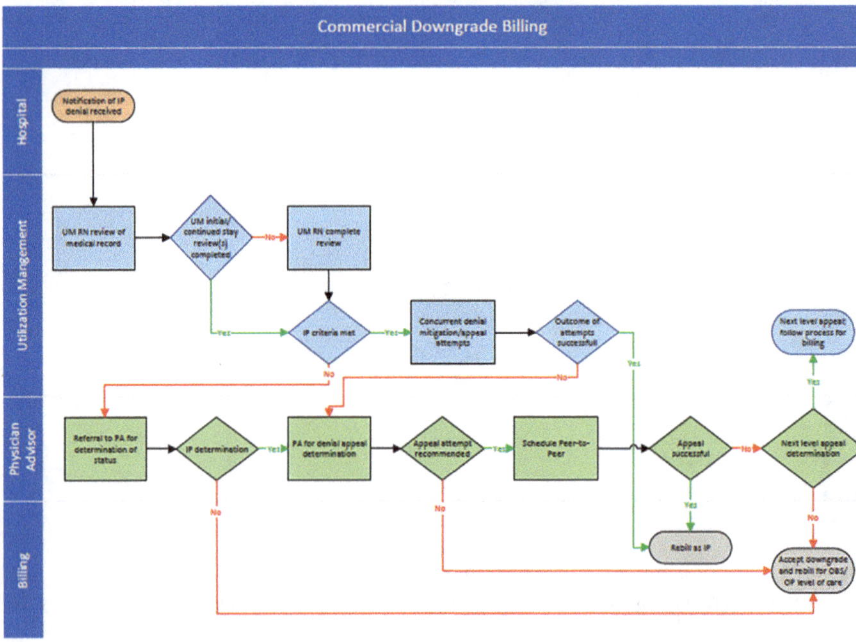

Fig. 9.14 A decision tree from the start of the process through the end as denoted by the oval shapes. Each diamond shape is a decision to be made following a yes or no pathway. Created by the author

Denial Management

See Fig. 9.15.

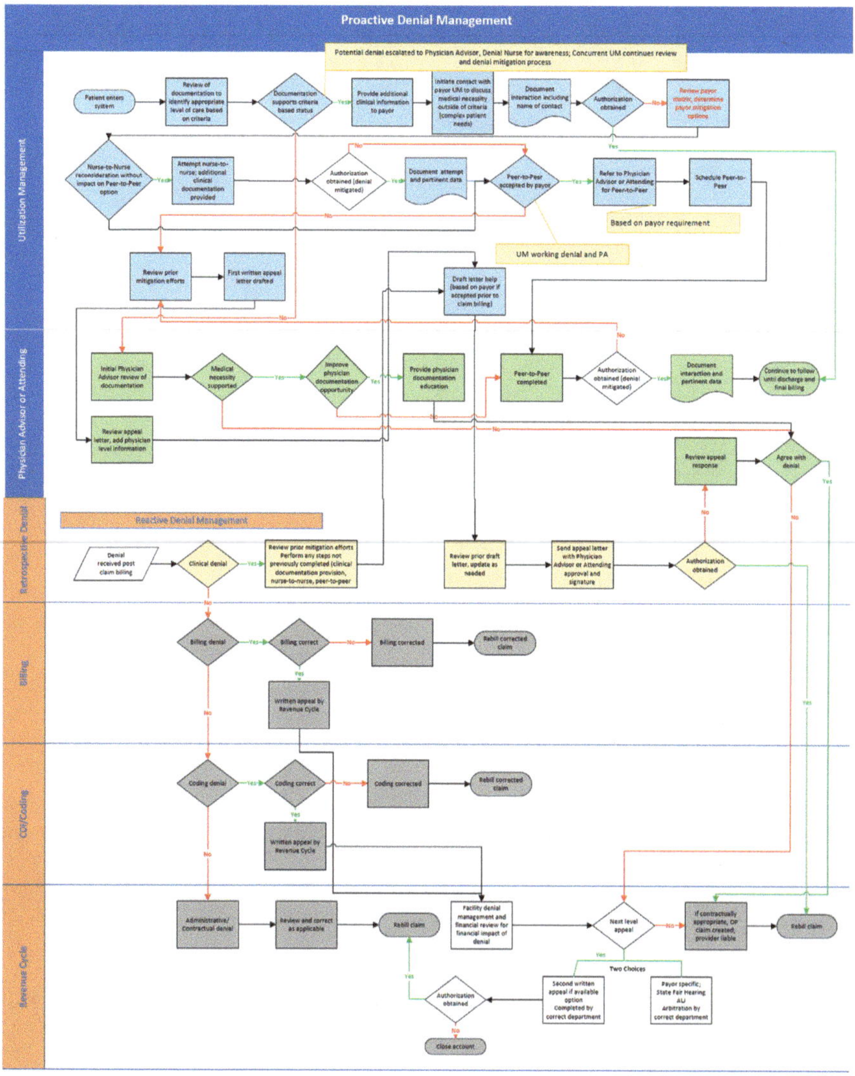

Fig. 9.15 A decision tree from the start of the process through the end as denoted by the oval shapes. Each diamond shape is a decision to be made following a yes or no pathway. Created by the author

Hospital-Issued Notice of Noncoverage (HINN 1)

See Fig. 9.16.

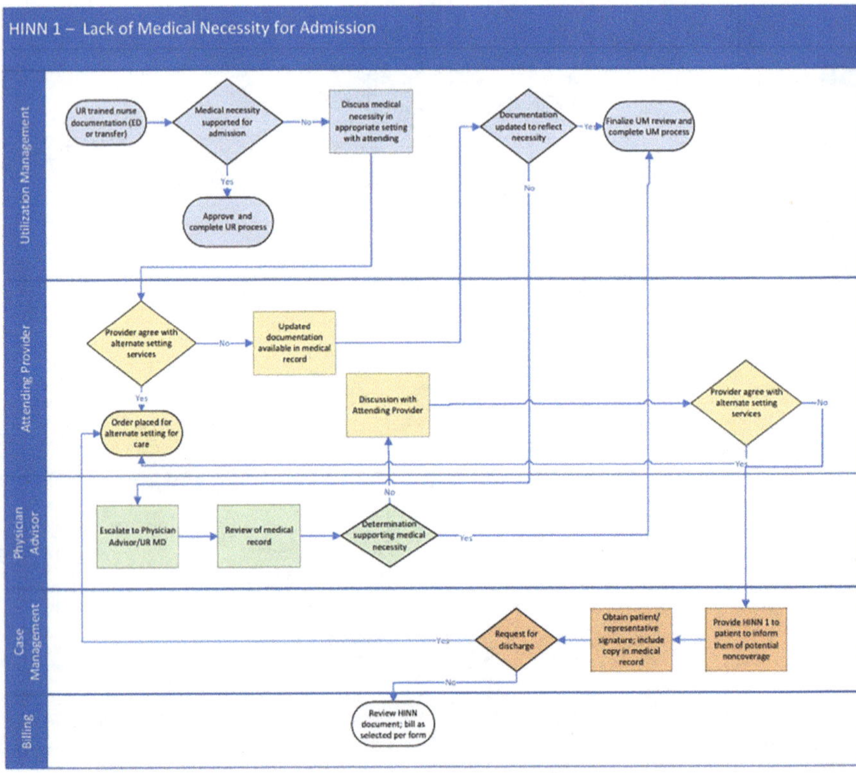

Fig. 9.16 A decision tree from the start of the process through the end as denoted by the oval shapes. Each diamond shape is a decision to be made following a yes or no pathway. Created by the author

Hospital-Issued Notice of Noncoverage (HINN 10)

See Fig. 9.17.

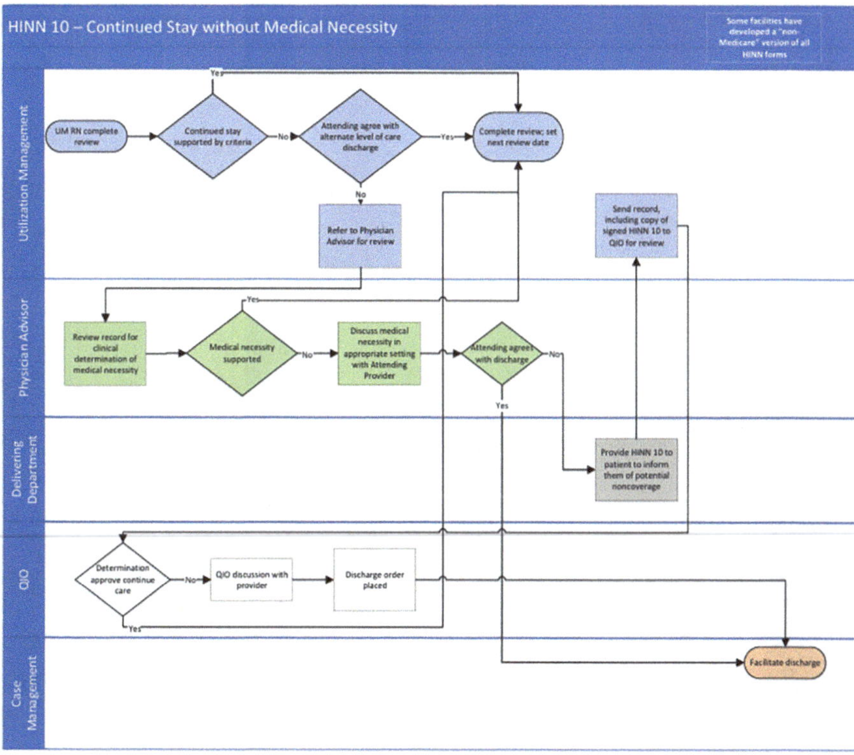

Fig. 9.17 A decision tree from the start of the process through the end as denoted by the oval shapes. Each diamond shape is a decision to be made following a yes or no pathway. Created by the author

Hospital-Issued Notice of Noncoverage (HINN 11)

See Fig. 9.18.

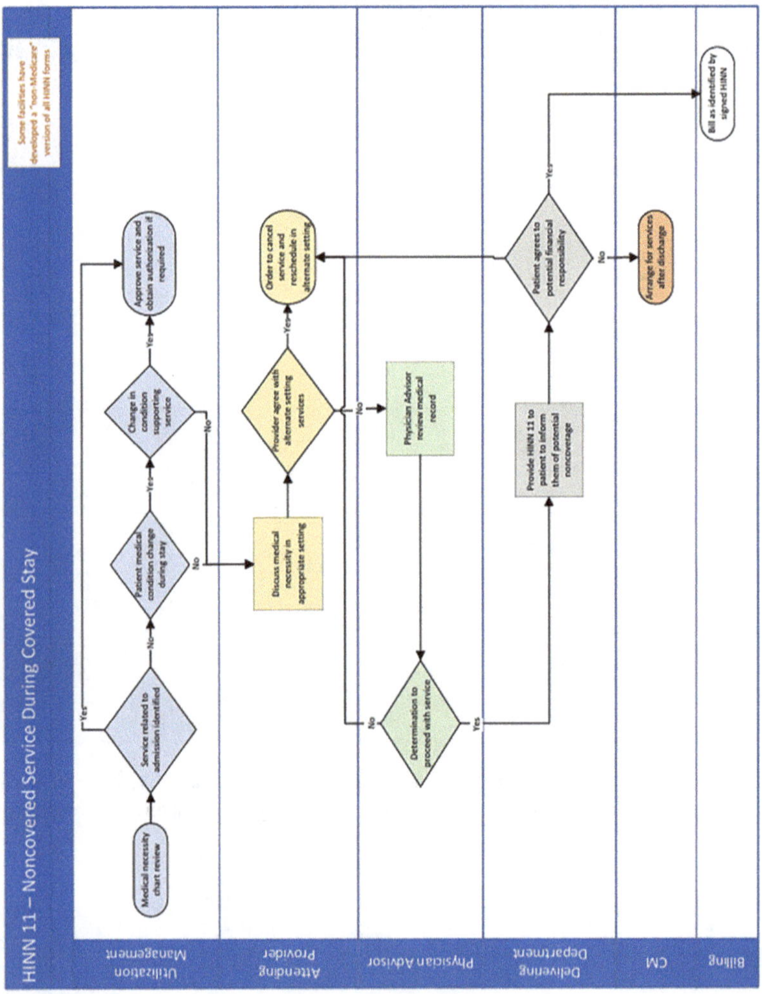

Fig. 9.18 A decision tree from the start of the process through the end as denoted by the oval shapes. Each diamond shape is a decision to be made following a yes or no pathway. Created by the author

Notice of Noncoverage (Not Acute Care Hospital Setting)

See Fig. 9.19.

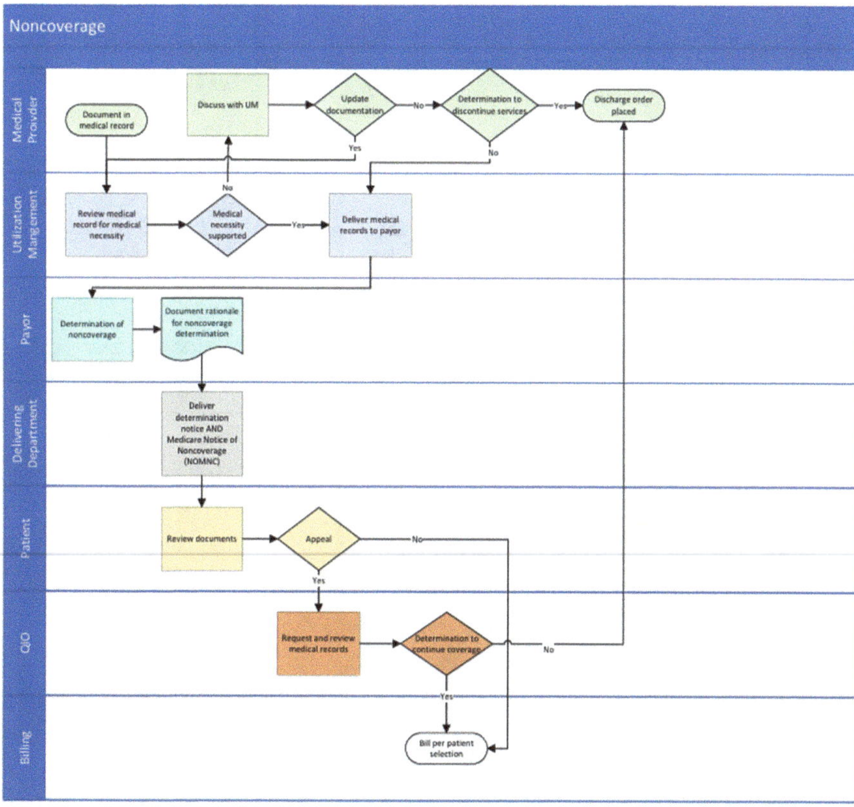

Fig. 9.19 A decision tree from the start of the process through the end as denoted by the oval shapes. Each diamond shape is a decision to be made following a yes or no pathway. Created by the author

QIO Request for Records

See Fig. 9.20.

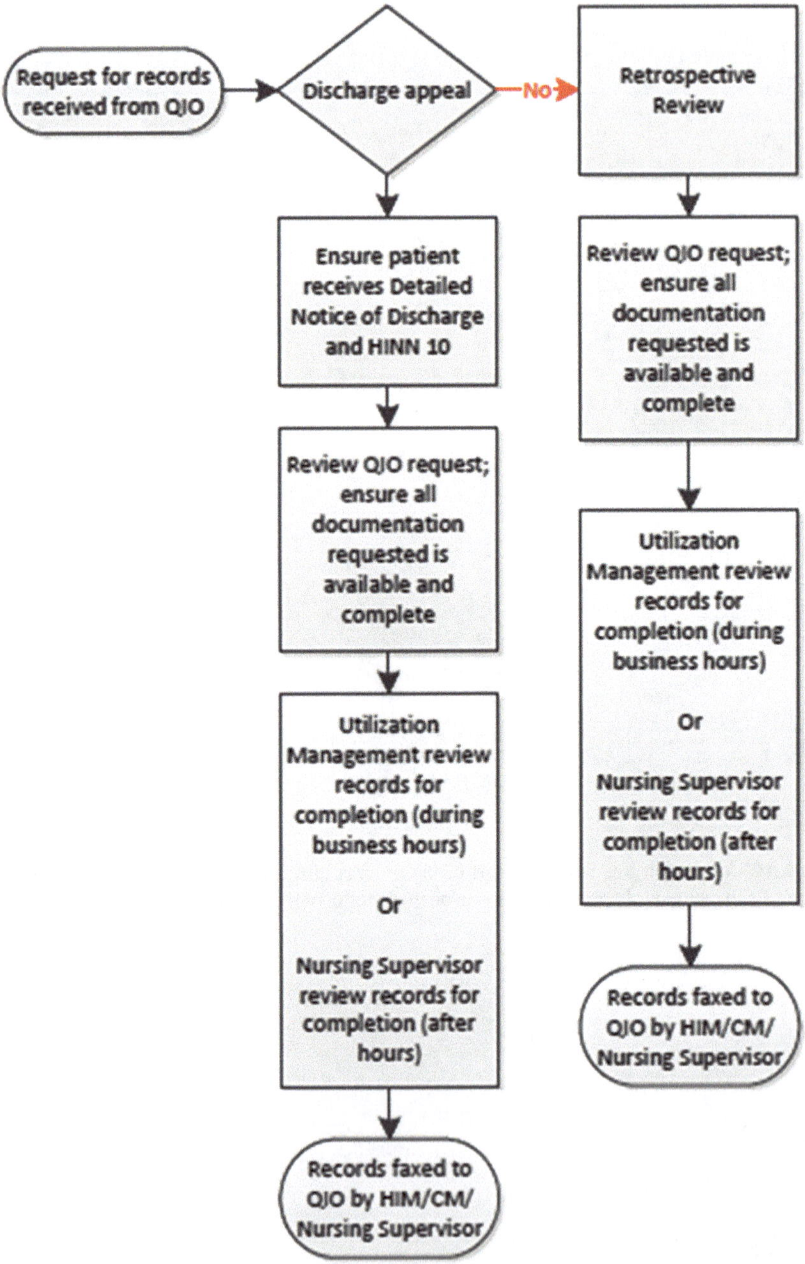

Fig. 9.20 A decision tree from the start of the process through the end as denoted by the oval shapes. Each diamond shape is a decision to be made following a yes or no pathway. Created by the author

9.3 Case Management Process Workflows

Many separate workflow processes apply to the Case Manager/Care Coordinator role. Again, it is important that UM and CM work closely together as much of the work is communicated in a two-way process for successful and compliant completion.

Important Message from Medicare (IMM)

See Fig. 9.21.

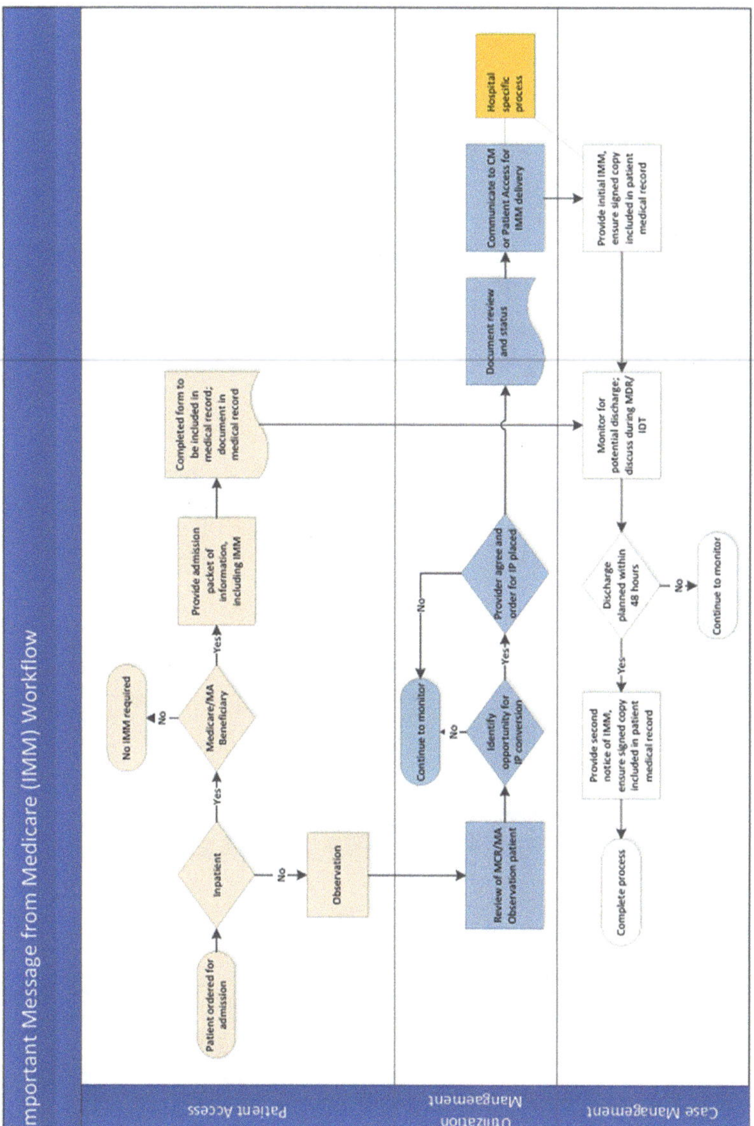

Fig. 9.21 A decision tree from the start of the process through the end as denoted by the oval shapes. Each diamond shape is a decision to be made following a yes or no pathway. Created by the author

Discharge Appeal

See Fig. 9.22.

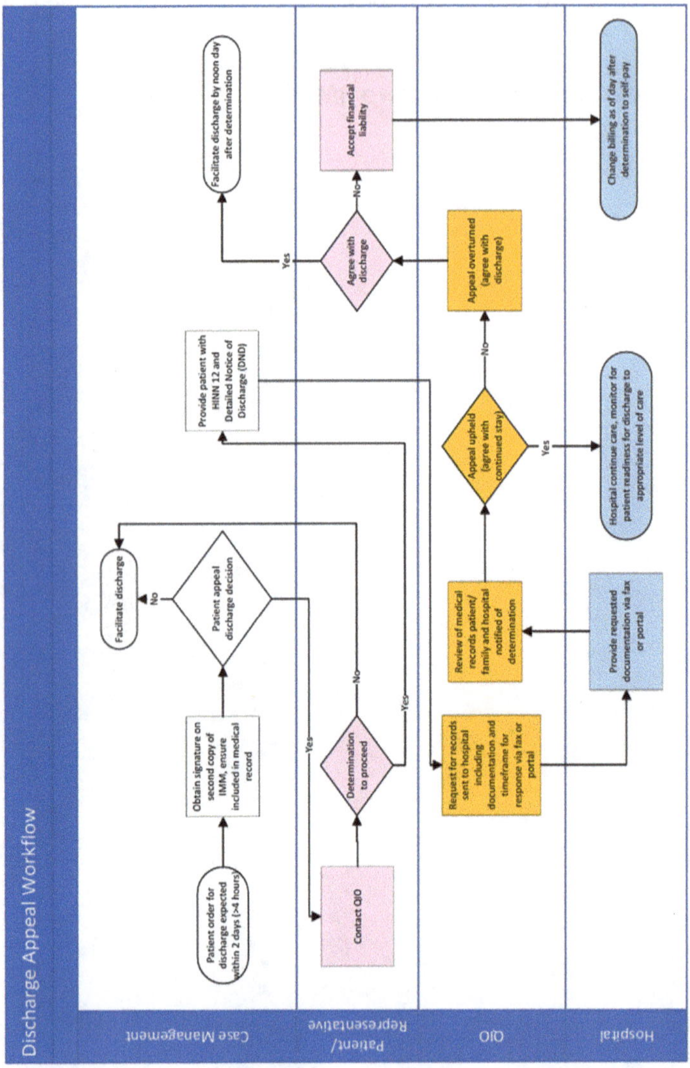

Fig. 9.22 A decision tree from the start of the process through the end as denoted by the oval shapes. Each diamond shape is a decision to be made following a yes or no pathway. Created by the author

9.4 Hospital-Issued Notice of Noncoverage (HINN 12)

See Fig. 9.23.

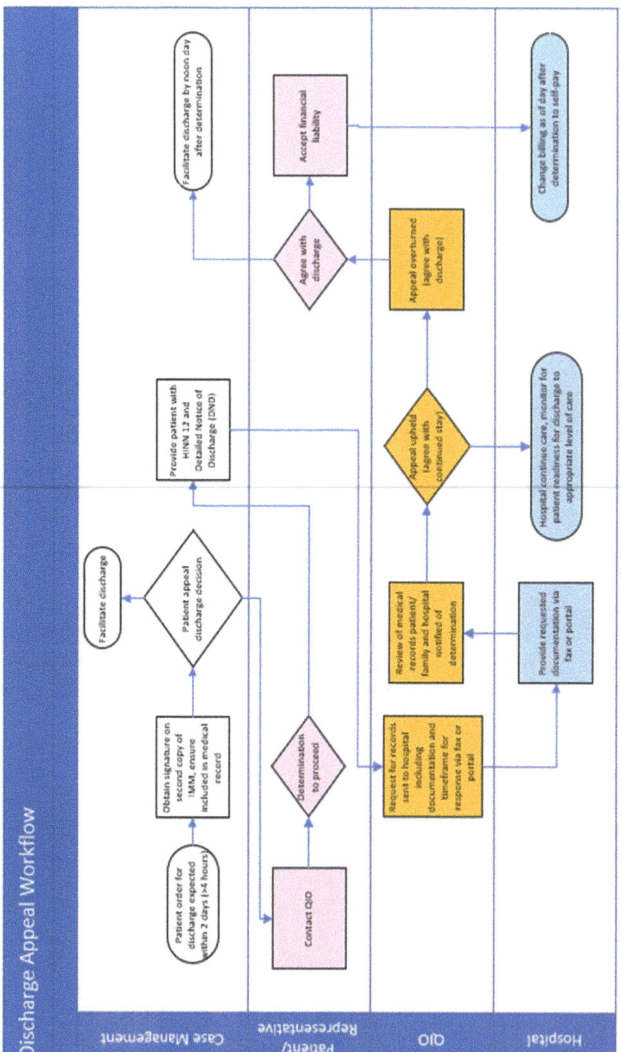

Fig. 9.23 A decision tree from the start of the process through the end as denoted by the oval shapes. Each diamond shape is a decision to be made following a yes or no pathway. Created by the author

High-Level CM Daily Process

See Fig. 9.24.

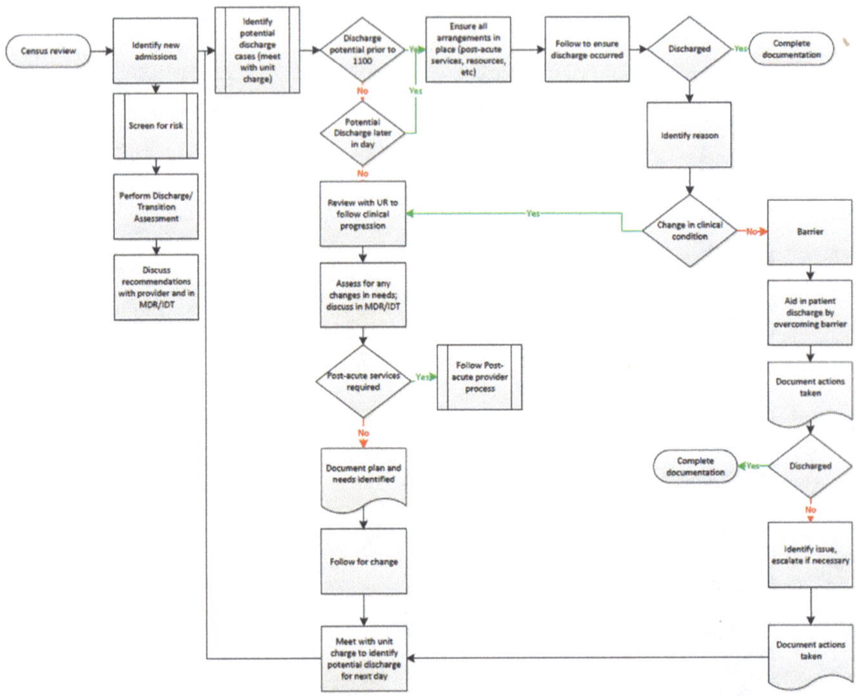

Fig. 9.24 A decision tree from the start of the process through the end as denoted by the oval shapes. Each diamond shape is a decision to be made following a yes or no pathway. Created by the author

Unfunded Patient Screening

See Fig. 9.25.

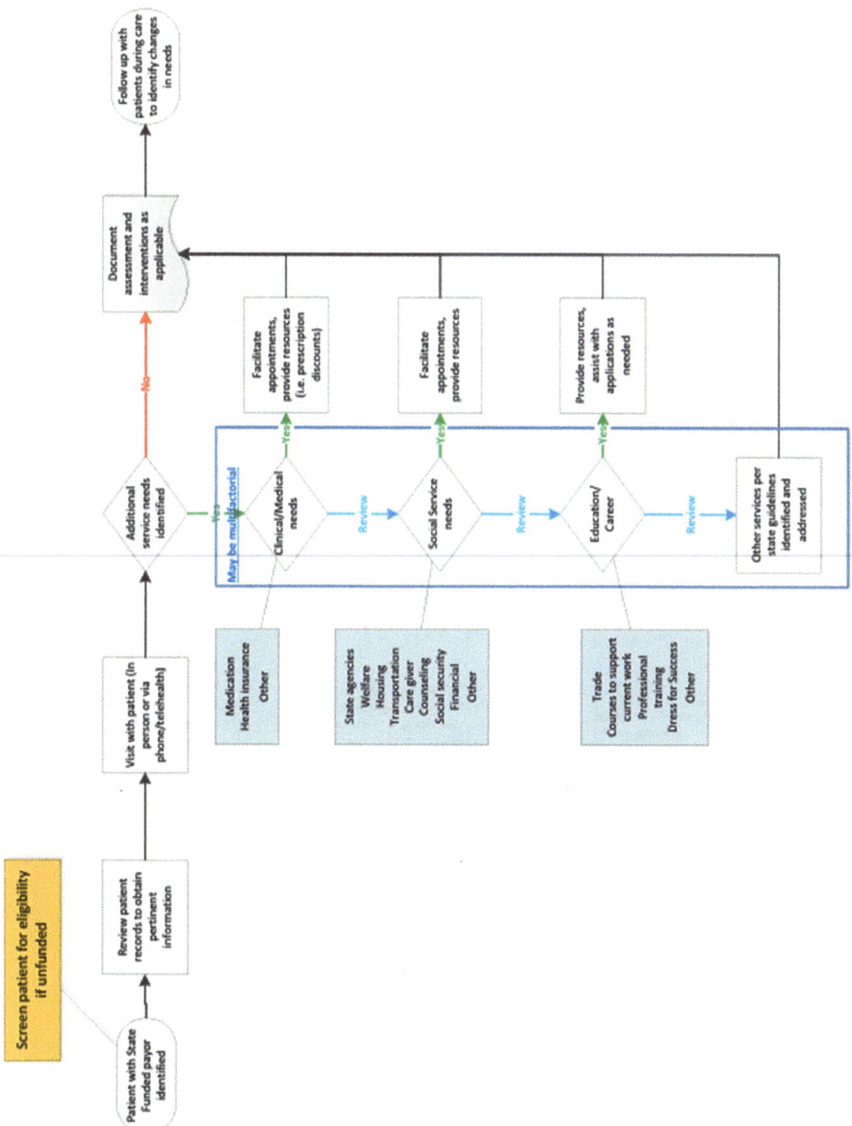

Fig. 9.25 A decision tree from the start of the process through the end as denoted by the oval shapes. Each diamond shape is a decision to be made following a yes or no pathway. Created by the author

Readmission Risk/Readmission Mitigation

See Fig. 9.26.

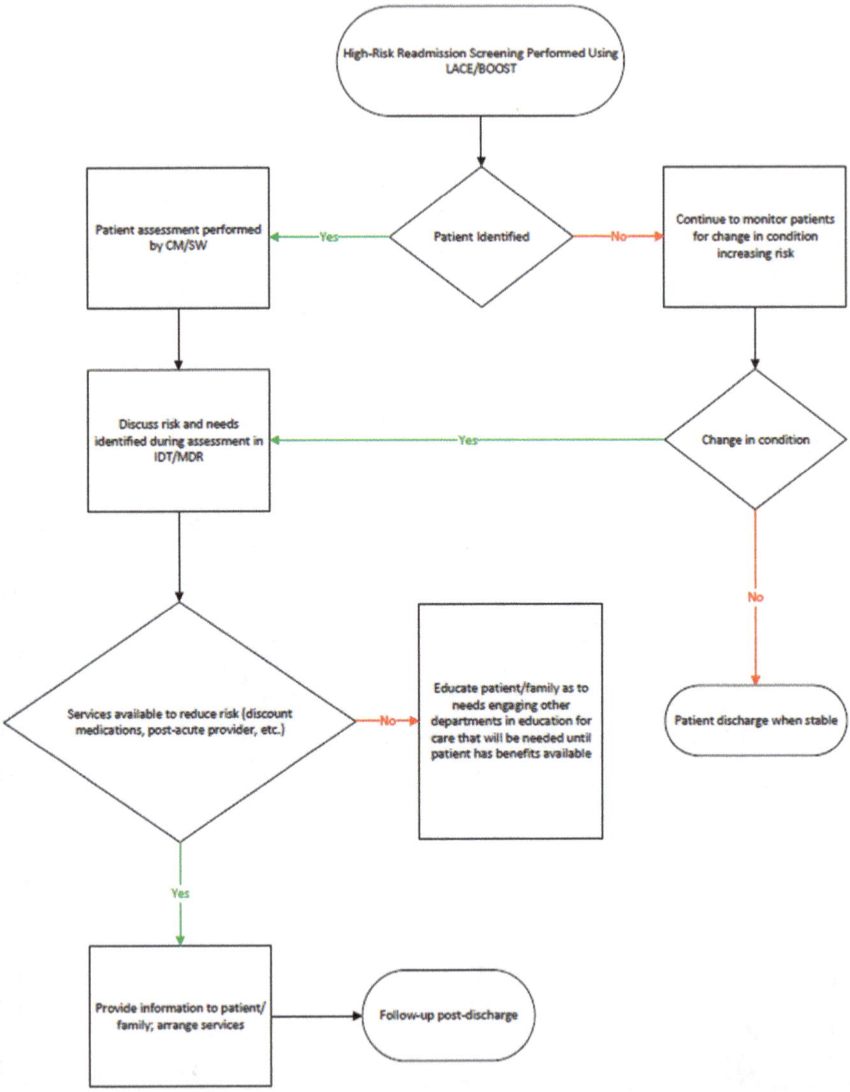

Fig. 9.26 A decision tree from the start of the process through the end as denoted by the oval shapes. Each diamond shape is a decision to be made following a yes or no pathway. Created by the author

Readmission Follow-Up

See Fig. 9.27.

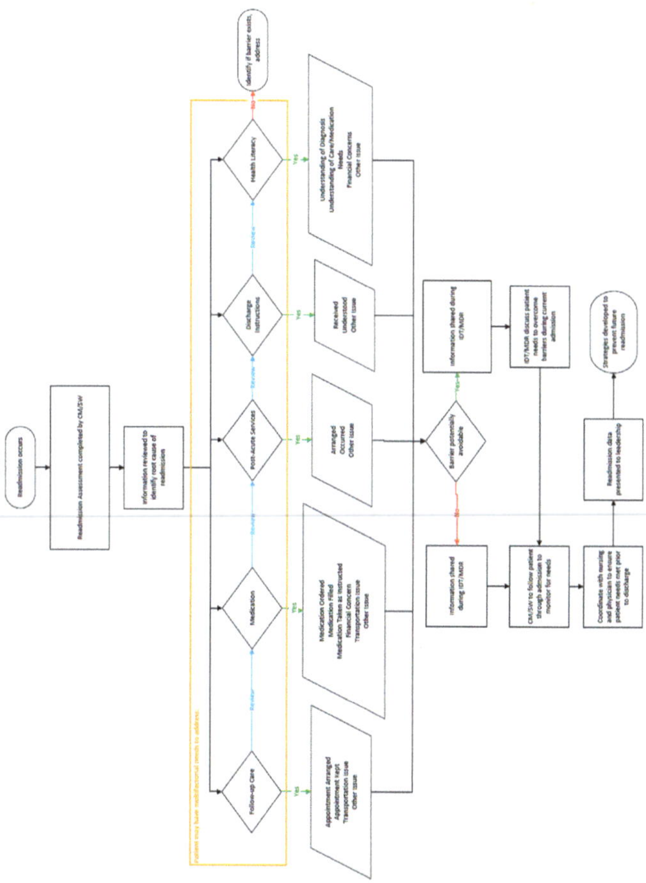

Fig. 9.27 A decision tree from the start of the process through the end as denoted by the oval shapes. Each diamond shape is a decision to be made following a yes or no pathway. Created by the author

Discharge Assessment

See Fig. 9.28.

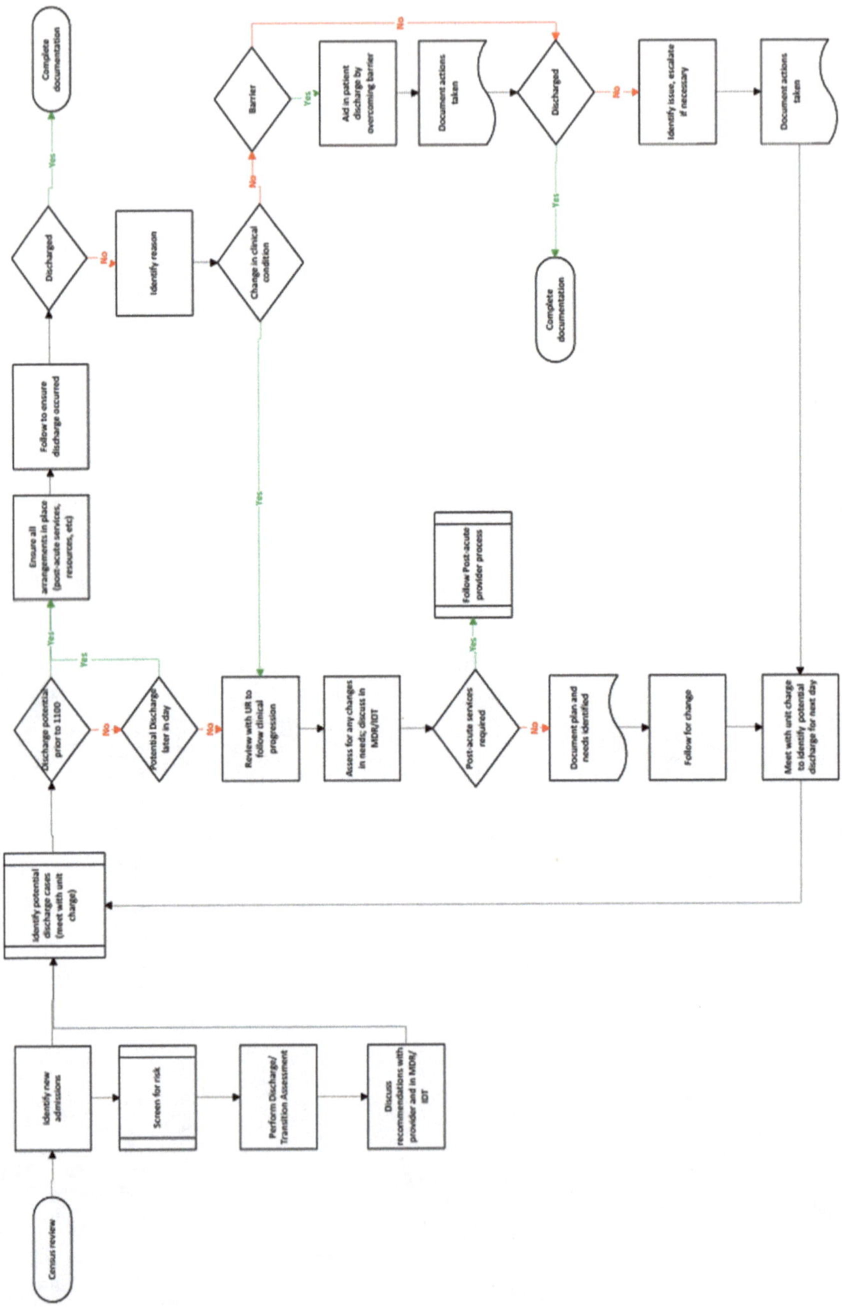

Fig. 9.28 A decision tree from the start of the process through the end as denoted by the oval shapes. Each diamond shape is a decision to be made following a yes or no pathway. Created by the author

Discharge Simple vs Complex

See Fig. 9.29.

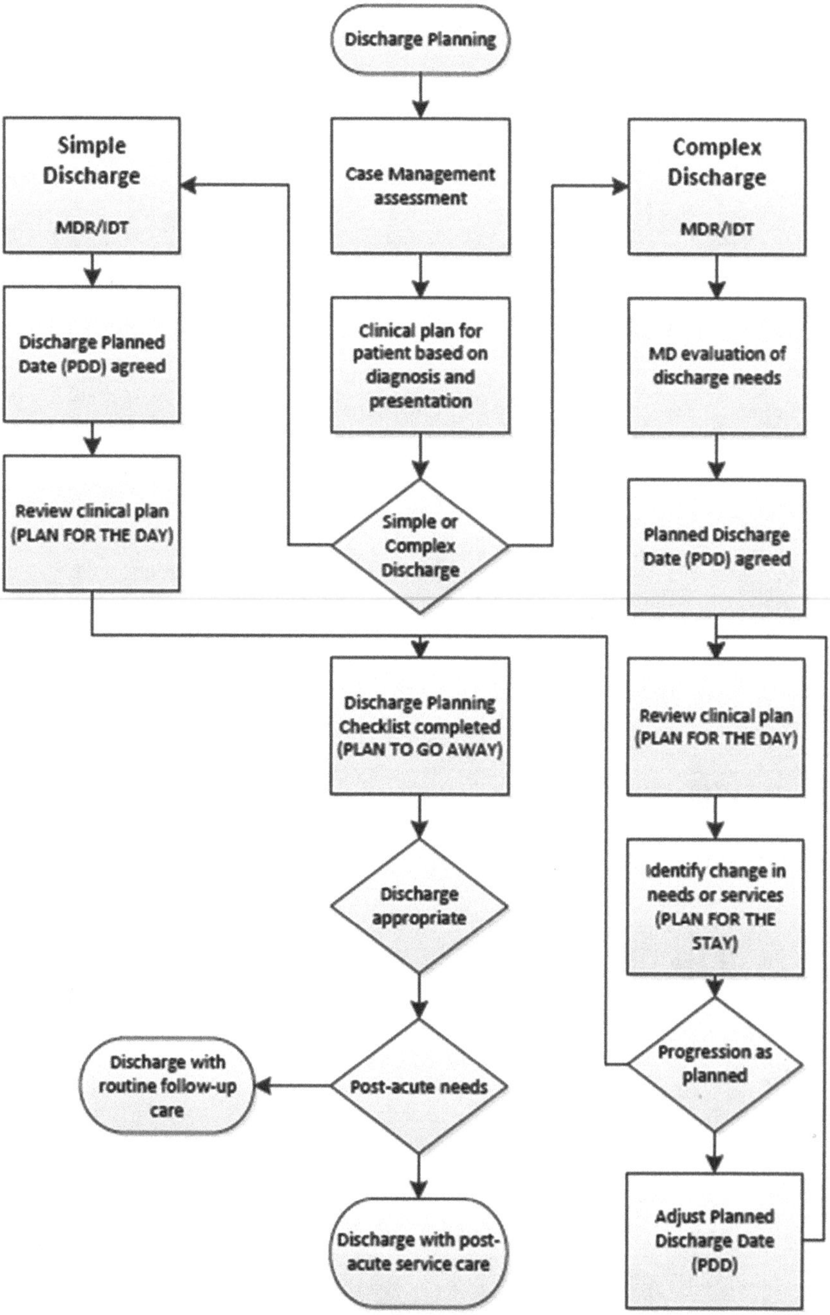

Fig. 9.29 A decision tree from the start of the process through the end as denoted by the oval shapes. Each diamond shape is a decision to be made following a yes or no pathway. Created by the author

Long-Stay High Risk Identification

See Fig. 9.30.

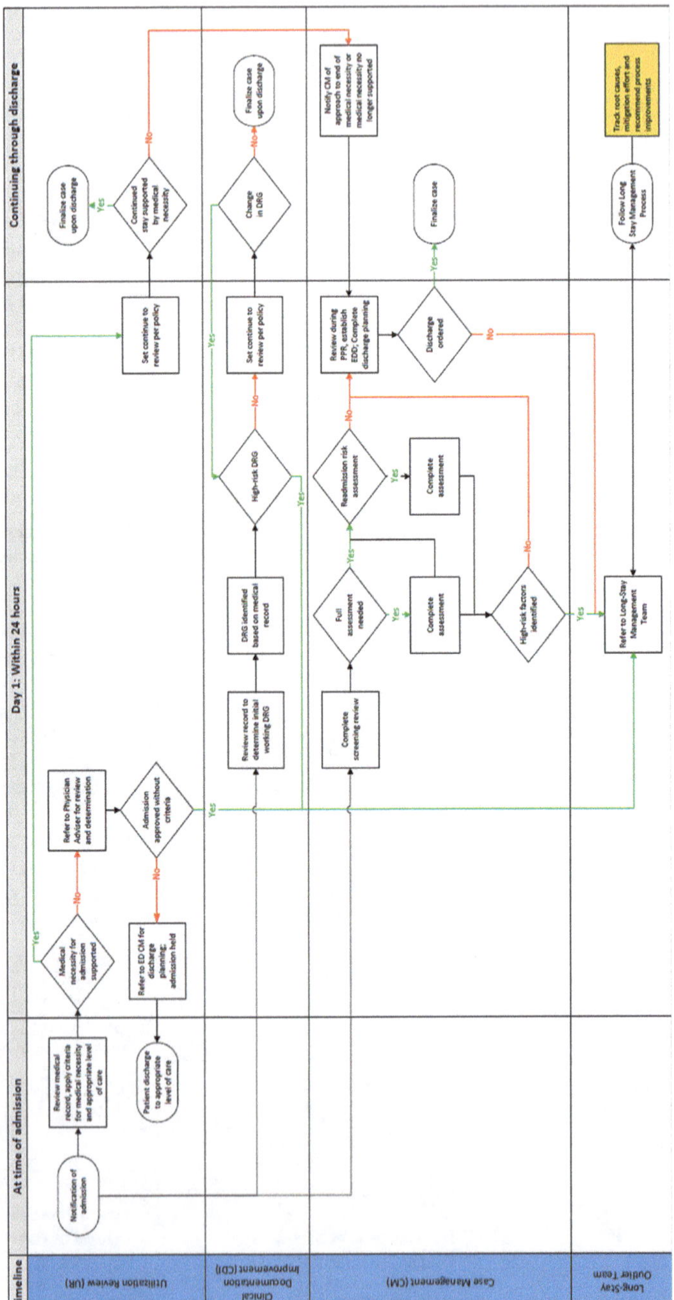

Fig. 9.30 A decision tree from the start of the process through the end as denoted by the oval shapes. Each diamond shape is a decision to be made following a yes or no pathway. Created by the author

MDR/PPR/IDT

See Fig. 9.31.

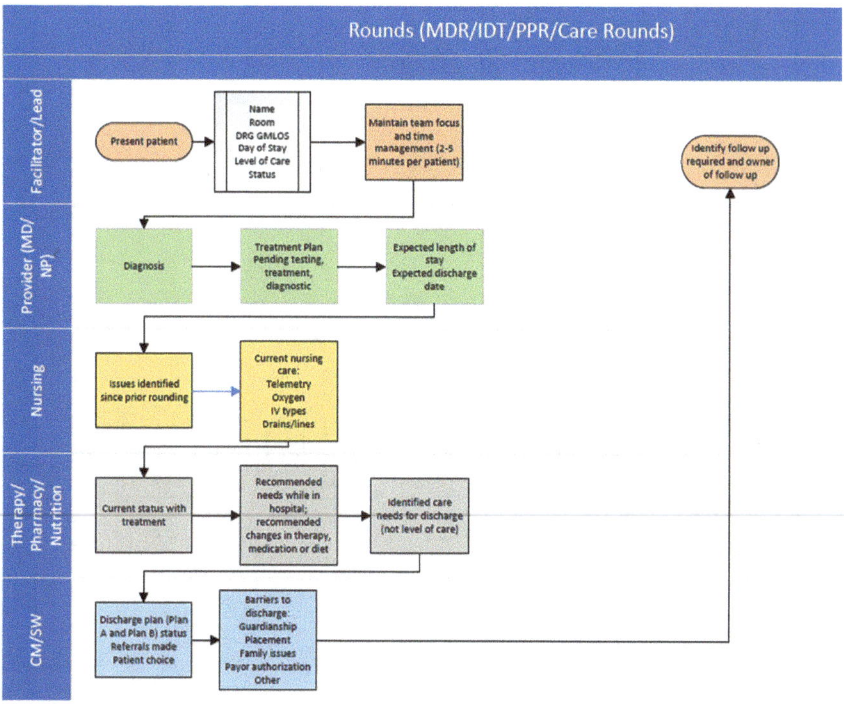

Fig. 9.31 A decision tree from the start of the process through the end as denoted by the oval shapes. Each diamond shape is a decision to be made following a yes or no pathway. Created by the author

Long-Stay Rounds

See Fig. 9.32.

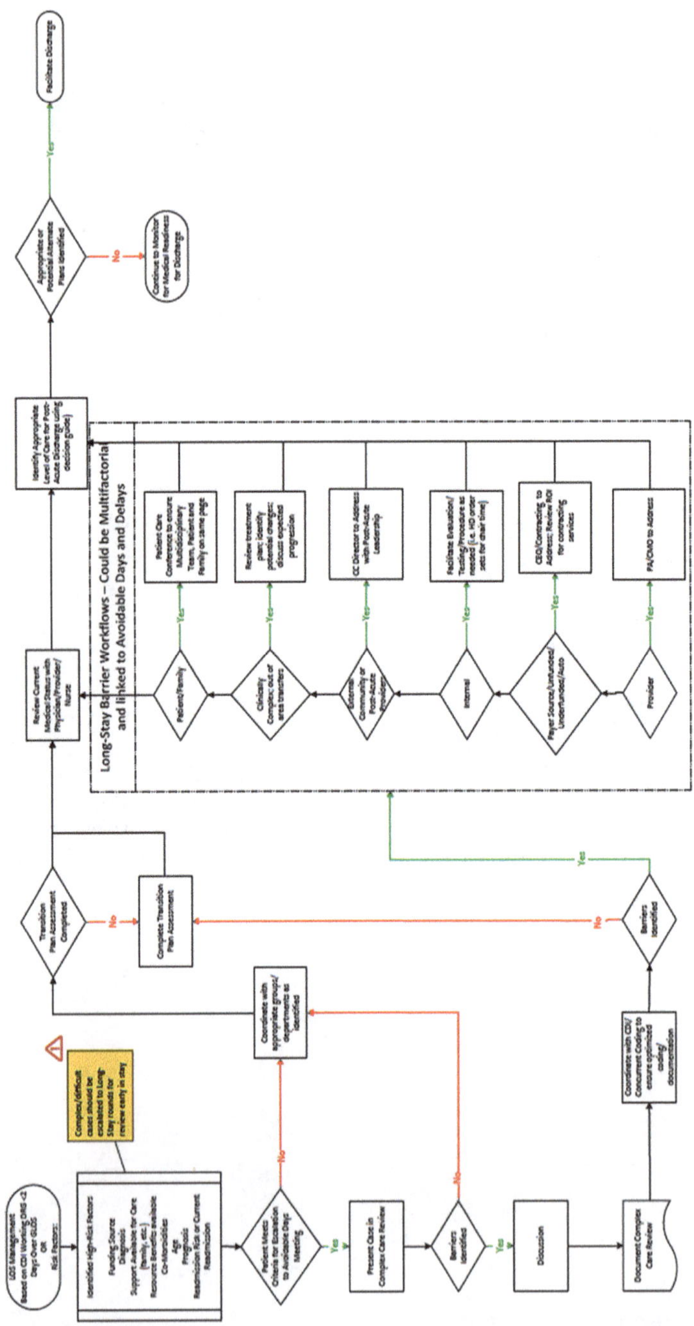

Fig. 9.32 A decision tree from the start of the process through the end as denoted by the oval shapes. Each diamond shape is a decision to be made following a yes or no pathway. Created by the author

Length of Stay Outlier—Non-Custodial

See Fig. 9.33.

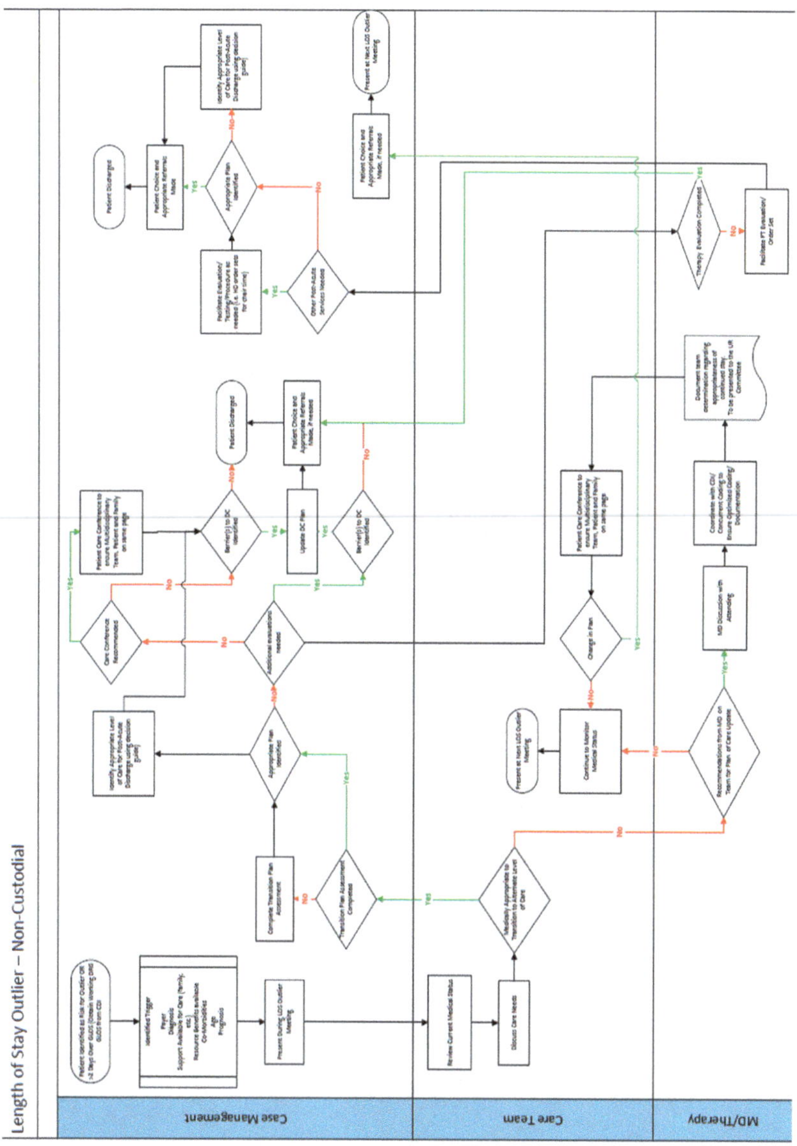

Fig. 9.33 A decision tree from the start of the process through the end as denoted by the oval shapes. Each diamond shape is a decision to be made following a yes or no pathway. Created by the author

Length of Stay Outlier—Custodial

See Fig. 9.34.

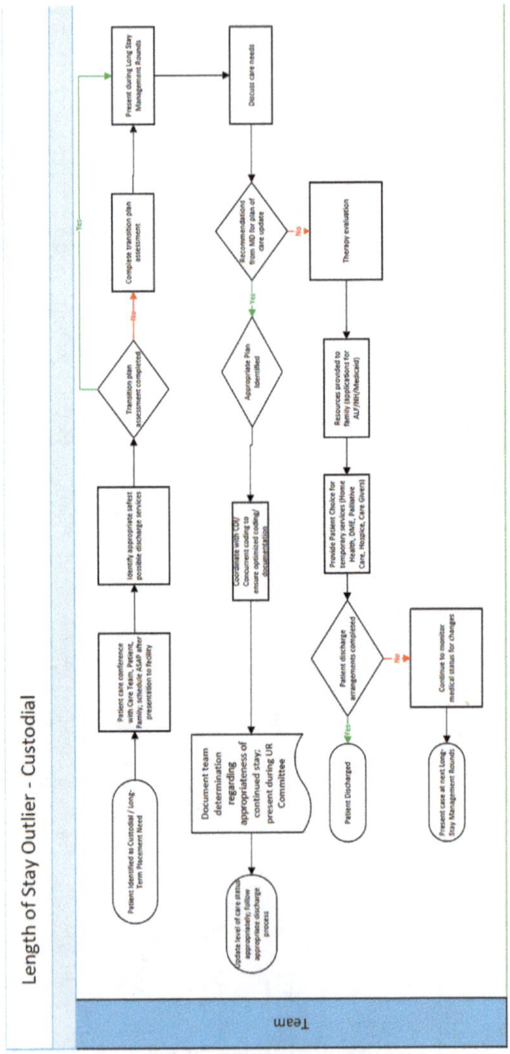

Fig. 9.34 A decision tree from the start of the process through the end as denoted by the oval shapes. Each diamond shape is a decision to be made following a yes or no pathway. Created by the author

Declining Discharge Escalation

See Fig. 9.35.

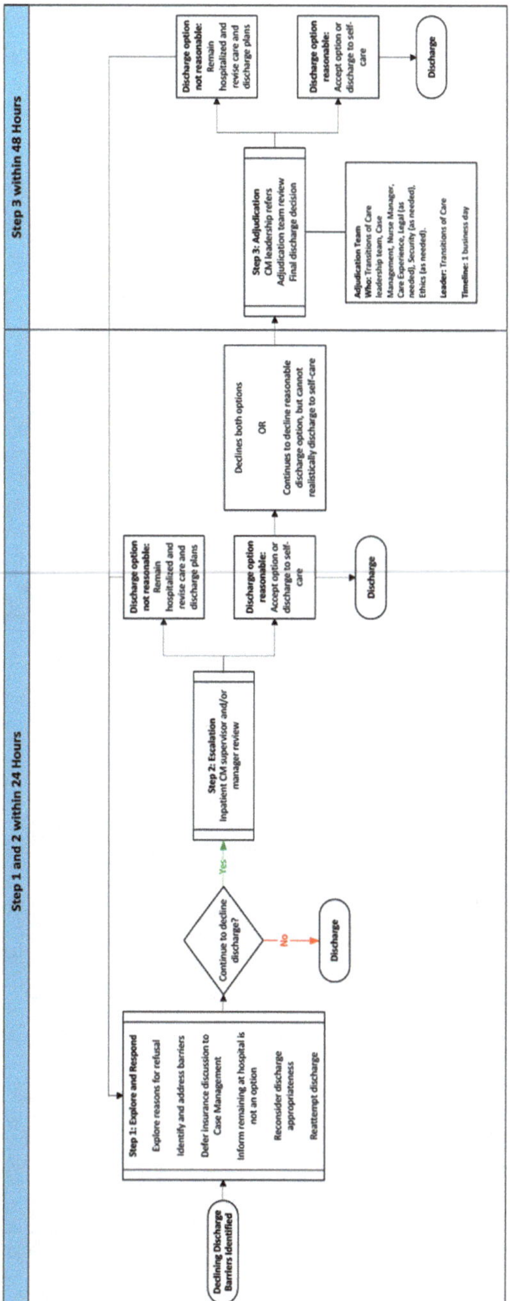

Fig. 9.35 A decision tree from the start of the process through the end as denoted by the oval shapes. Each diamond shape is a decision to be made following a yes or no pathway. Created by the author

Post-Acute Provider Discharge

See Fig. 9.36.

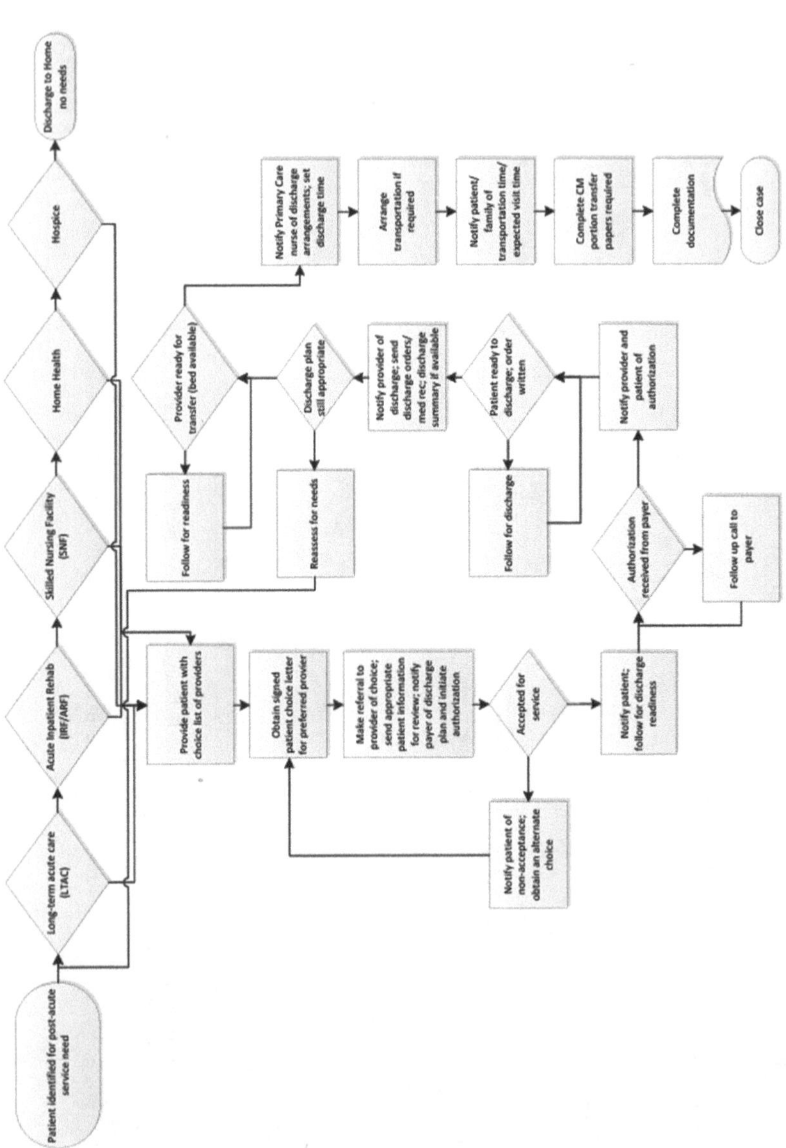

Fig. 9.36 A decision tree from the start of the process through the end as denoted by the oval shapes. Each diamond shape is a decision to be made following a yes or no pathway. Created by the author

Transitional Care

See Fig. 9.37.

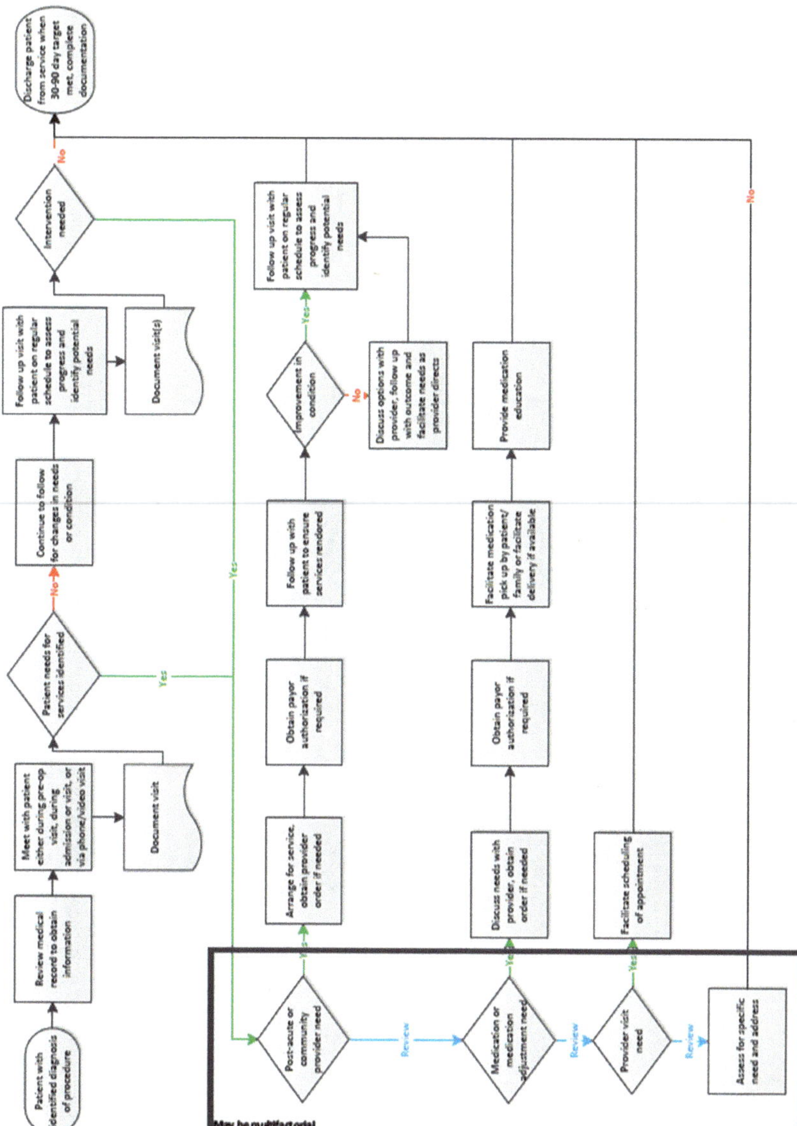

Fig. 9.37 A decision tree from the start of the process through the end as denoted by the oval shapes. Each diamond shape is a decision to be made following a yes or no pathway. Created by the author

Avoidable Delay/Day High-Level

See Fig. 9.38.

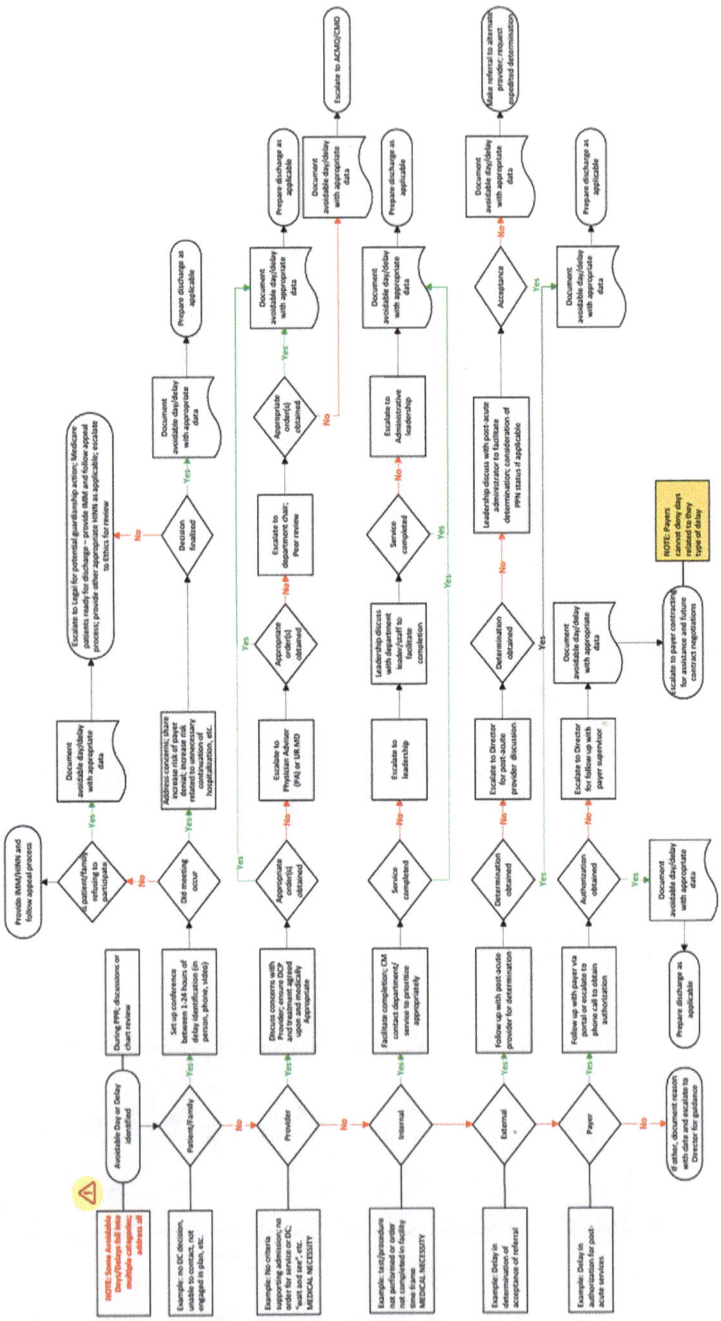

Fig. 9.38 A decision tree from the start of the process through the end as denoted by the oval shapes. Each diamond shape is a decision to be made following a yes or no pathway. Created by the author

Avoidable Delay—Patient or Family Barrier

See Fig. 9.39.

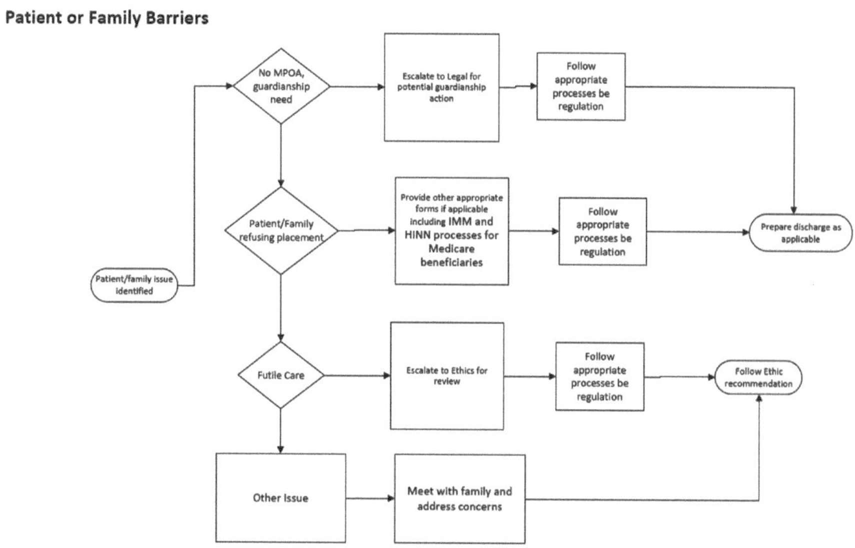

Fig. 9.39 A decision tree from the start of the process through the end as denoted by the oval shapes. Each diamond shape is a decision to be made following a yes or no pathway. Created by the author

Avoidable Delay Potential—Complex Care

See Fig. 9.40.

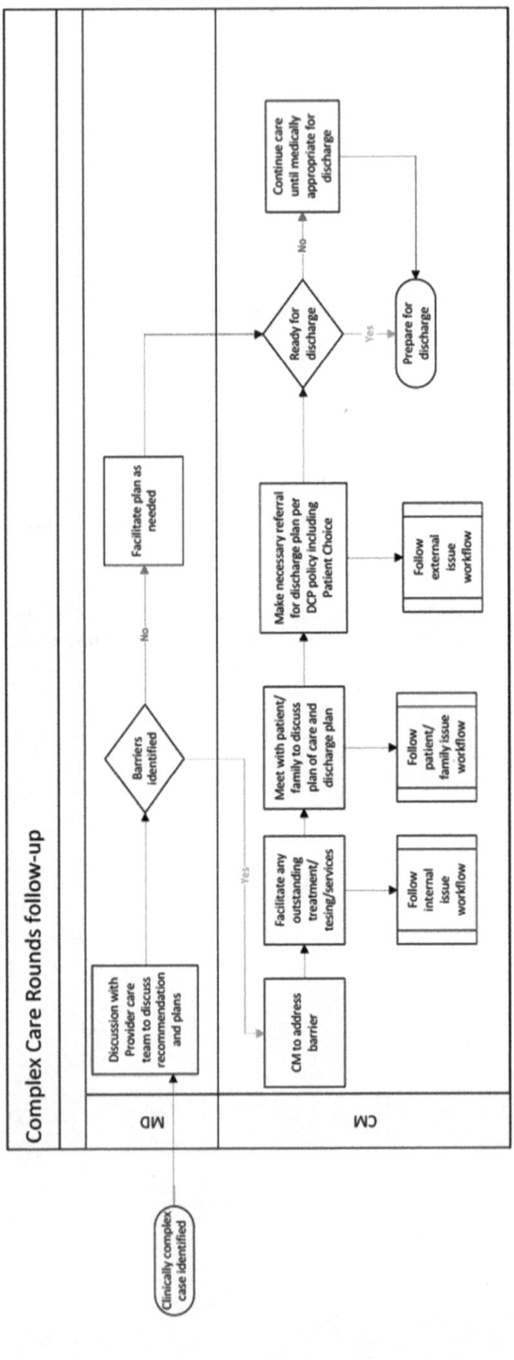

Fig. 9.40 A decision tree from the start of the process through the end as denoted by the oval shapes. Each diamond shape is a decision to be made following a yes or no pathway. Created by the author

Avoidable Delay/Day—External

See Fig. 9.41.

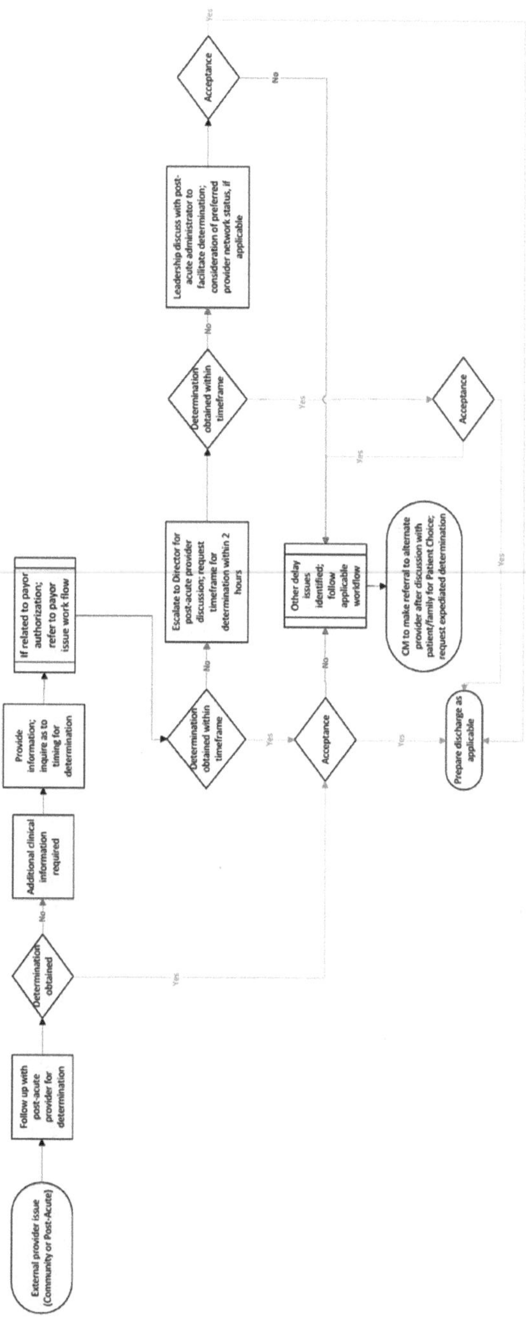

Fig. 9.41 A decision tree from the start of the process through the end as denoted by the oval shapes. Each diamond shape is a decision to be made following a yes or no pathway. Created by the author

Avoidable Delay/Day—Internal

See Fig. 9.42.

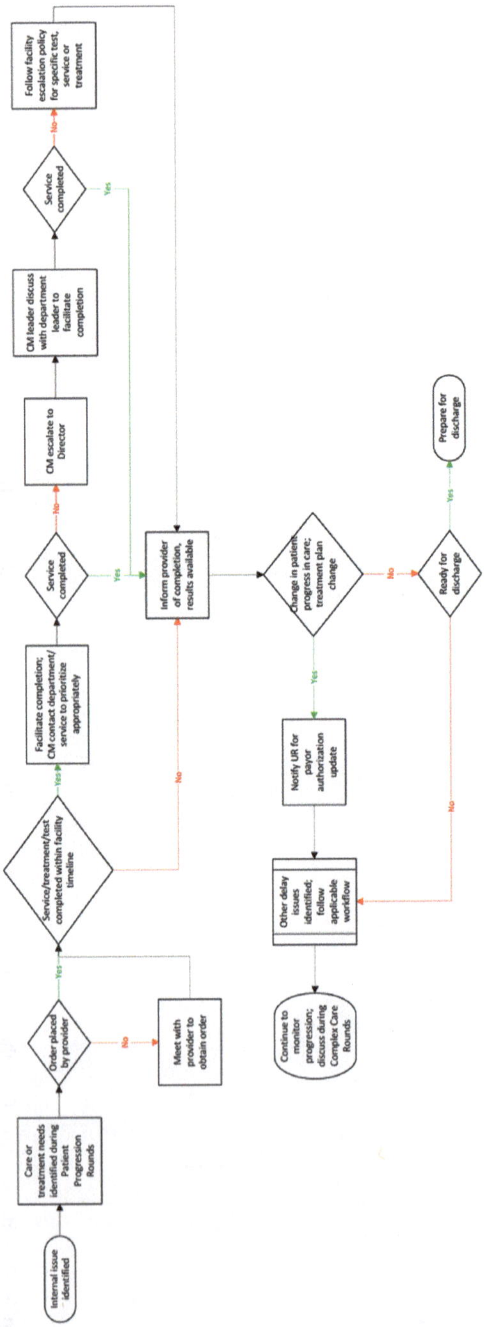

Fig. 9.42 A decision tree from the start of the process through the end as denoted by the oval shapes. Each diamond shape is a decision to be made following a yes or no pathway. Created by the author

Avoidable Delay/Day—Provider

See Fig. 9.43.

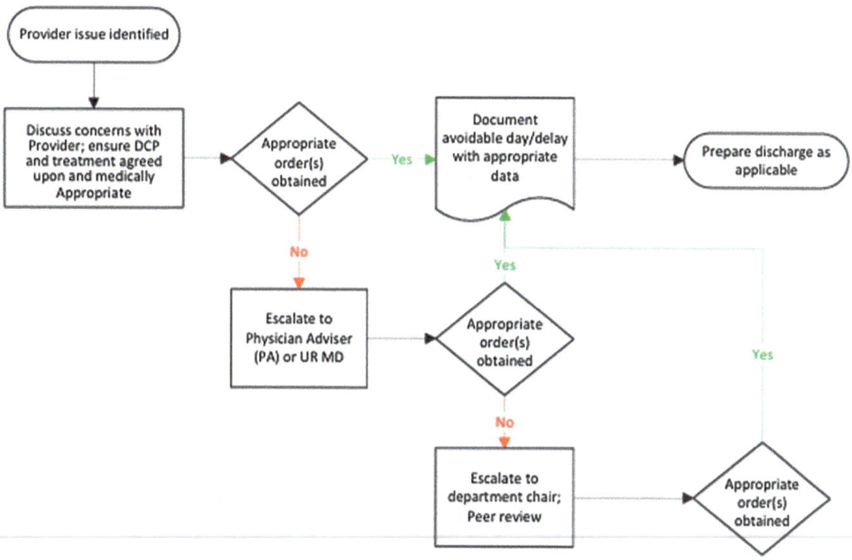

Fig. 9.43 A decision tree from the start of the process through the end as denoted by the oval shapes. Each diamond shape is a decision to be made following a yes or no pathway. Created by the author

Avoidable Delay/Day—Payor

See Fig. 9.44.

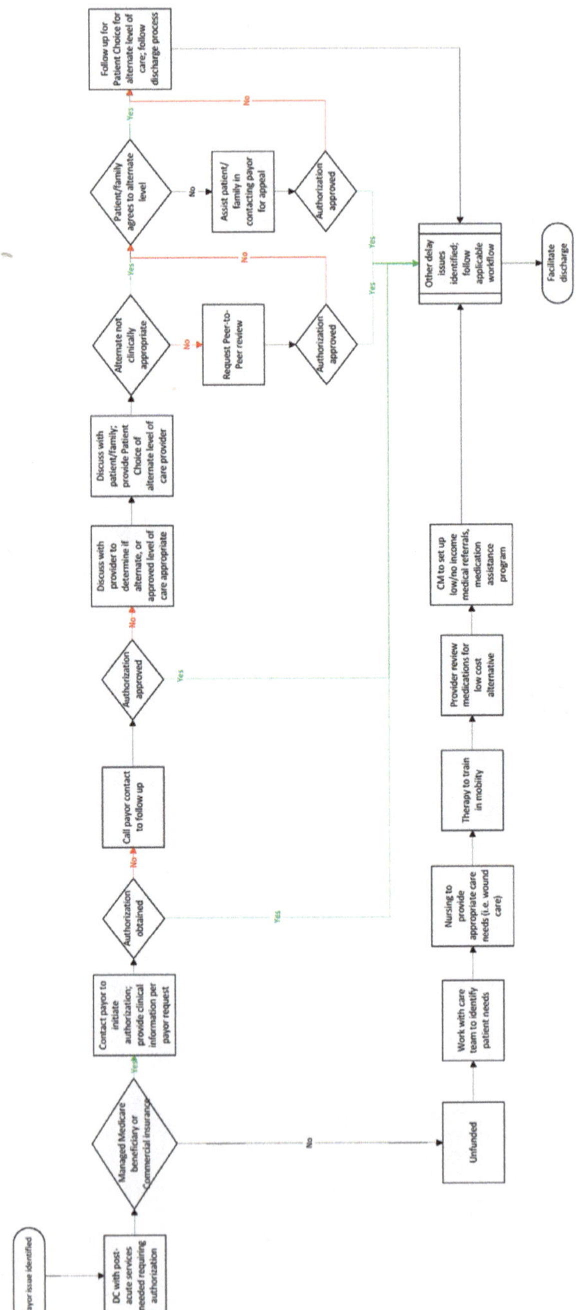

Fig. 9.44 A decision tree from the start of the process through the end as denoted by the oval shapes. Each diamond shape is a decision to be made following a yes or no pathway. Created by the author

10 Educational Tip Sheets

Learning Objectives

1. **Implement Best Practices:** Foster knowledge of best practices in healthcare that can optimize operations and resource management, ultimately leading to higher patient satisfaction rates.
2. **Promote Continuous Improvement:** Inspire a culture of continuous improvement by utilizing easily digestible resources that keep healthcare providers informed and engaged in maintaining high-quality care.

In the ever-evolving landscape of healthcare, it is crucial for providers and organizations to stay informed about regulations, best practices, and essential guidelines. The healthcare environment is impacted by numerous factors, including changes in legislation, advancements in medical technology, and shifts in patient expectations. Therefore, healthcare professionals must be equipped with up-to-date knowledge to ensure they can deliver the highest quality care while remaining compliant with legal standards.

This section provides a collection of Tip Sheets designed to offer concise and valuable insights into key areas crucial for effective healthcare delivery. These areas include Conditions of Participation, which outline the minimum standards that healthcare facilities must meet to participate in Medicare and Medicaid programs; Conflict of Interest policies that ensure transparency and integrity in clinical decision-making; and Utilization Management practices that focus on the appropriate use of healthcare resources.

These resources serve as practical tools for healthcare professionals to navigate the complex compliance requirements that characterize today's healthcare landscape. The Tip Sheets condense important information into a format that is easily accessible, enabling practitioners to reference them in their daily operations without wading through dense legal texts or lengthy documents.

S. Garceau, *Interdisciplinary Case Management: A Nursing Practice Approach*,
https://doi.org/10.1007/978-3-032-20960-3_10

By understanding fundamental concepts through these Tip Sheets, healthcare providers can ensure they are consistently aligned with regulatory standards. This alignment is not only beneficial from a compliance standpoint but is also integral to enhancing patient care. Improved knowledge and adherence to guidelines can lead to better patient outcomes, reducing hospital readmission rates, minimizing medical errors, and fostering a culture of safety and quality in healthcare delivery.

As healthcare organizations strive for excellence, utilizing these resources can also support organizational success. Providers and administrators who are aware of best practices can implement changes that optimize operations, improve resource management, and ultimately lead to higher patient satisfaction rates.

These Tip Sheets are more than just informational resources; they are vital instruments for inspiring continuous improvement within healthcare settings. By distilling important information into easily digestible formats, they empower healthcare providers to remain informed, compliant, and committed to delivering exceptional care to their patients.

10.1 Conditions of Participation (CoP) Tip Sheet

Centers for Medicare and Medicaid Services (CMS) requires providers and suppliers of healthcare to abide by the Conditions of Participation to receive reimbursement for services. This includes hospitals, home health, hospice and nursing homes and the services for treatment, therapy services and diagnosis services of patients. CMS-approved accrediting organizations such as The Joint Commission and DNV monitor compliance.

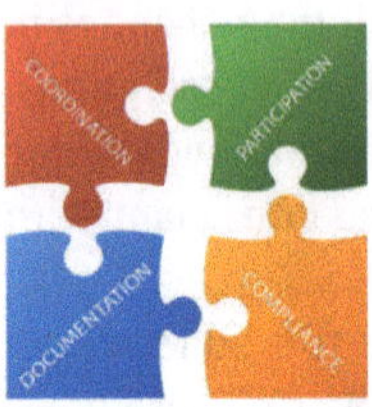

> The Conditions of Participation were established to align state licensure requirements and declare minimal health and safety requirements across healthcare providers throughout the country.

The four key elements included in the Conditions of Participation. Created by the author

What Are the Conditions of Participation?

CMS developed qualifications that healthcare organizations must meet in order to begin and continue participating in federally funded health care programs including Medicare, Medicaid, CHIPS, etc. These standards involve health and safety guidelines that protect all beneficiaries by improving quality and enforcing patient rights. The Conditions of Participation apply to all healthcare organizations.

What Conditions of Participation Apply to Utilization Management?

- Utilization review for medical necessity and use of patient benefits including scope and frequency of reviews
- Review of professional services provided to patients are in the correct setting
- Physician Advisor program
- Utilization Management Committee oversight
- Extended stay reviews
- Patient rights related to notices: Condition Code 44, Occurrence Span Code 72, delivery of Important Message from Medicare (IMM) or Medicare Outpatient Observation Notice (MOON) and Medicare Notice of Status Change (MNSC) when status changes during the admission; Hospital Issued Notice of Noncoverage (HINN) as applicable to the services provided in the incorrect setting
- Confidentiality of patient records
- Performance improvement initiatives for department

What Is the Value of the Conditions of Participation?

Improved compliance	Improved patient safety
Protection of patient rights	Support hospital revenue
Improved quality of care	Standards of care maintained

10.2 Conflict of Interest Tip Sheet

Financial conflict of interest MUST be disclosed to patients within the hospital, including, but not limited to a hospital provider has a financial interest or ownership in a Home Health Services provider.

We are obligated to share any potential conflict of interest to patients or their representative. This will allow the patient to make a choice without pressure to select a specified provider but are giving full disclosure in order to make an educated decision.

What Is Considered Conflict of Interest?

Conflict of interest definitions are codified in four federal policy initiatives: The Balancing Incentive Program within The Affordable Care Act (ACA); Community First Choice (CFC) within the ACA; Home and Community-Based Services (HCBS) Settings Final Rule (CMS 2249F) and The Older Americans Act Reauthorization Act.

CMS has defined Case Management Conflict of Interest (COI) as:

- When the same entity helps an individual gain access to services *and* provides services to that individual.
- When the same entity is responsible for assuring and honoring free choice of providers *and* is a service provider.

What Is the Stark Law?

- It must be disclosed to patients if the physician, or his family member, has a financial involvement in the post-acute provider they are recommending.
- Remember, Patient MUST ALWAYS receive choice. Even if the payor source only covers one provider, if the patient requests, more choices are offered.
- Use a wide range of vendors. If you are part of an Accountable Care Organization in your area, and you have preferred providers you work with in order to meet the requirements, you must disclose this to the patient, and if they request other providers, those must be offered.
- A violation of the Conflict-of-Interest federal regulation can lead to a job loss and federal prosecution.

What Is the Value of the Reviewing Conflict of Interest?

Compliance with CMS Honor patient choice
Allow patients to make an educated decision

10.3 Utilization Management Committee Tip Sheet

CMS Condition of Participation §482.30 states "determination of medical necessity for admission or continued stay rests with the admitting physician or member of the UR committee or subgroup thereof."

Did you know the UR Committee is the only committee required by the Medicare Conditions of Participation and must report through to the Medical Executive Committee to the Board of Directors?

Who Are the Participants of the UR Committee?

2 Physicians **REQUIRED**	Chief Financial Officer	Chief Nursing Officer
UM/CM Directors	Quality Department	Risk Management
Health Information Management	Patient Access	

Department Directors from patient care units

How Often and Where Does the UR Committee Meet?

Per Condition of Participation, UR Committee is required to meeting at a minimum on a quarterly basis however, best practice is for a monthly meeting of the URC.

What Does the UR Committee Discuss?

Analytics	Readmission cases	Financial reporting
Avoidable/denied days	RAC audits	Case studies
PA referrals	Discharge disposition	Patient follow-up

Information and minutes from the Utilization Review Committee are shared with the Medical Executive Committee and the facility Board of Directors.

What Is the Value of the Utilization Review Committee?

Compliance with Conditions of Participation	Increased satisfaction
Improved quality of care	Improved patient experience
Improved coordination of teamwork	Process improvement identification

10.4 Two-Midnight Rule Tip Sheet

On October 30, 2015, CMS released updates to the Two-Midnight rule regarding when Inpatient admissions are appropriate for payment under Medicare Part A. These changes continue CMS' long-standing emphasis on the importance of the physician's medical judgment in meeting the needs of Medicare beneficiaries.

Inpatient admissions are considered reasonable and necessary for Medicare beneficiaries who require more than a 1-day stay in the hospital or who need treatment specified as inpatient only.

How Was the Two-Midnight Rule Developed?

Review of Recovery Audit Program (RAC), CMS identified high rates of error for hospital services rendered in a medically unnecessary setting (i.e., Inpatient rather than Outpatient).

Observed higher frequency of beneficiaries being treated as hospital outpatients and receiving extended observations services.

What Is the Basic Principle of the Two-Midnight Rule?

The admitting physician expects that patient to require hospital care that crosses two midnights.

Based on complex medical factors such as patient history and comorbidities, the severity of signs and symptoms, current medical needs, and the risk of an adverse event.

Clinical expectation must be documented in the medical record.

Hospital must monitor to ensure that a physician's decision to admit a beneficiary is supported by clear documentation in the patient's medical record.

Inpatient admission for surgical procedure specified by Medicare as "Inpatient Only" as the guideline.

Are There Exclusions from the Two-Midnight Rule?

Transfer to another acute care facility, transition to hospice or palliative care, Against Medical Advice discharge, patient expires, initiation of mechanical ventilation, and those.

How Are Audits Viewed By CMS?

Review for documentation regarding need for admission and patient condition. One day stay review to determine Inpatient Only procedure, exclusion criteria, previous midnight in Observation status and physician documentation as to medical necessity.

What Is the Value of the Two-Midnight Rule?

Compliance with CMS	Increased patient satisfaction
Mitigate recoupment penalties	Mitigate denials
Improve bed management	Improve resource utilization

10.5 Condition Code 44 (CC44) Tip Sheet

CMS Condition of Participation §482.30 (d), states "Be sure to understand Medicare rules and policy when Utilization Review (UR) determines that an Inpatient admission is not medically necessary or when a hospital should report Condition Code 44 on Outpatient claims to signal a change in patient status from Inpatient to Outpatient."

Per the Conditions of Participation §482.13, require a hospital to protect and promote each patient right including the right to be notified regarding the change in status impacting the patient's financial liability

What Are Documentation Requirements for a CC 44?

All orders and all entries related to the Inpatient admission must be retained in the record in their original form. Patient's status change must be fully documented in medical record.

What Must Be Considered Prior to a CC 44?

Change made PRIOR to discharge, while the beneficiary is still a patient of the hospital No Inpatient claim has been submitted to Medicare.

What Are the Steps for the Physician and Facility in the CC 44 Process?

- Inpatient status order placed in patient record
- UM review with criteria application does not support Inpatient level of care, discussion with attending to obtain additional documentation, re-review for criteria supported documentation, if not:
- Referral to Physician Advisor for review for clinical judgement of medical necessity, PA determination Inpatient is not supported
- PA discussion with attending regarding documentation improvement and status change to Observation
- Attending agrees with Observation, UM Committee MD added to conversation with PA and attending for concurrence of attending and at least one other physician for status
- If concurrence is for Observation appropriate status correction, attending documents in medical record and enters Observation order, AND UM notifies CM to delivery Medicare Outpatient Observation Notice (MOON) to patient as well as the Medicare Notice of Status Change (MNSC) and patient's right to appeal
- Documentation completed by CM of delivery of notice
- Case reported during UM Committee meeting

What Is the Value in a Condition Code 44?

Compliance with Conditions of Participation	Decreased denial rates
Increased communication	Increased patient satisfaction

10.6 Occurrence Span Code 72 Tip Sheet

To ensure accurate tracking of the Two-Midnight requirement for inpatient level of care, CMS allows hospitals to use the Occurrence Span Code 72 to track outpatient care prior to inpatient admission.

Previously, the inpatient claim only allowed CMS to track inpatient time after a patient was formally admitted as an inpatient. Using the Occurrence Span Code 72 allows providers and review contractors to identify the total number of midnights on the face of the claim (inpatient and observation).

> Occurrence Span Code 72 identifies, and reports outpatient services received within a short time frame before an inpatient admission

How Does Utilization Management Identify Accounts to Be Billed with Occurrence Code 72?

Using a standard screening process for all short stay accounts will provide a method for the Utilization Management department to identify case with treatment supporting the addition of Occurrence Span Code 72 to be added to billing. These cases are excluded from the PEPPER "one day stay" report as these patient meet the requirement to meet the expectancy for length of time receiving hospital level of care services as part of the Two-Midnight Rule.

What Services Count Towards an Occurrence Span Code 72?

Time spent receiving services in:	
Emergency department	Observation services
Time spent at a transferring facility	Outpatient treatment area services

What Is the Value of the Occurrence Span Code 72?

Improved billing compliance	Decrease denials
Improve revenue	Improve resource utilization

10.7 Important Message from Medicare (IMM) Tip Sheet

Per CMS-4105-F, "hospitals are required to deliver the Important Message from Medicare (IM), CMS-R-193 to all Medicare beneficiaries who are admitted to the hospital Inpatient level of care, including those with Medicare as a secondary payor. If the beneficiaries choose to appeal a discharge decision, they must receive the Detailed Notice of Discharge (DND) CMS 10066."

All hospitals that are paid under the Inpatient Prospective Payment (IPPS) are required to follow the Important Message and Appeal of Discharge process

Who Received the Important Message from Medicare Notices?

ALL Medicare and Medicare Advantage beneficiaries.

What Is the Important Message from Medicare and Detailed Notice of Discharge?

The Important Message from Medicare is a hospital Inpatient admission notice given to all beneficiaries with Medicare, Medicare and Medicaid (dual-eligible), and Managed Medicare. This is a notification to the beneficiary of their right to appeal the discharge decision. The Detailed Notice of Discharge is designed to give the patient further explanation about why the hospital and/or physician believe that the medical services are no longer necessary.

When Do These Notices Need to Be Given?

CMS guidelines state that the initial copy of the Important Message from Medicare be given to the patient, or representative, within 2 calendar days of admission to Inpatient status. The second copy of the notice is given prior to discharge, **NOT MORE than 2 days prior** to discharge, and **AT LEAST 4 h before** the time of discharge. CMS strongly recommends a signature or initials of the patient/representative be obtained on follow-up notice, although it is not required, documentation is required that the second notice was provided to the beneficiary or representative.

What Role Does Case Management/Utilization Management Play in the Process?

Case Management is a patient and facility advocate in the IMM and DND process. Case Management follows the patient from admission through discharge and can track those patients requiring these notifications. Provide the follow-up notice is **NOT** required for patients who are transferred from one Inpatient hospital setting to another Inpatient hospital setting.

What Is the Value of the Important Message?

Compliance with Conditions of Participation
Ensure patient rights are protected

10.8 Medicare Outpatient Observation Notice (MOON) Tip Sheet

The MOON is a standardized notice to inform beneficiaries (including Medicare health plan enrollees) that they are an outpatient receiving observation services and are not an inpatient of the hospital or critical access hospital (CAH).

The MOON is mandated by the Federal Notice of Observation Treatment and Implication for Care Eligibility Act (NOTICE Act), passed on August 6, 2015. All hospitals and CAHs are required to provide the MOON beginning no later than March 8, 2017.

The NOTICE Act requires hospitals and CAHs to provide notification to individuals receiving observation services as outpatients for more than 24 h explaining the status of the individual as an outpatient, not an inpatient, and the implications of such status.

What Is Considered Outpatient Observation Services?

- Services provided to help your doctor decide if you need to be admitted as an Inpatient or discharged from the hospital.
- Given in the Emergency Department or another areas of the hospital.
- Usually last 48 h or less.

Are There Guidelines for the Notification?

- Must be delivered to beneficiaries in Original Medicare (fee-for-service) and Medicare Advantage enrollees who receive observation services as outpatients for more than 24 h and no later than 36 h after observation services as an outpatient begin.
- The statute expressly provides that the MOON be delivered to beneficiaries who receive **observation** services as an outpatient for more than 24 h.
- Intended to inform beneficiaries receiving observation services for more than 24 h that they are outpatients receiving observation services and not inpatients, and the reasons for the status,
- Hospitals and CAHs may deliver the MOON to an individual receiving observation services as an outpatient *before* the 24 h mark has been reached.

- An explanation of the MOON must be provided, ideally in conjunction with the delivery of the notice, and a signature must be obtained from the patient or representative, to acknowledge receipt. In cases where such individual or person refuses to sign the MOON, the staff member should document refusal to sign.
- Electronic issuance of the MOON is permitted.

What Is Covered in Under the Medicare Outpatient Observation Notice?

Informing patient that stay is not covered under Medicare Part B, including:

- A copayment for each outpatient hospital service received.
- Copyaments vary by type of service.
- Medicare Part A requires a 3-day, medically necessary, Inpatient admission if Skilled Nursing Facility (SNF) care is needed after hospital stay.

What Is the Value of MOON?

Maintain Medicare compliance	Improve patient satisfaction
Mitigate denials	Improve communication
Education regarding appropriate status	

10.9 Hospital-Issued Notice of Noncoverage (HINN) Tip Sheet

Hospitals provide Hospital-Issued Notice of Noncoverage (HINN) to beneficiaries prior to admission, at admission, or at any point during an Inpatient stay, if the hospital determines that the care the beneficiary is receiving, or is about to receive, is not covered because it is: (1) not medically necessary; (2) not delivered in the most appropriate setting, or (3) is custodial in nature.

HINN 1	For those cases being referred for Inpatient admission without medical necessity: custodial services, convenience prior to surgery/procedure, etc.
HINN 10	Case not meeting medical necessity for continued stay and physician not agreeing with discharge. Cases being denied by Managed Medicare due to medical necessity and facility determines admission is appropriate
HINN 11	Testing unrelated to hospital admission being ordered for convenience of provider or patient
HINN 12	Patient has appealed their discharge, the HINN 12 is provided in addition to the Detailed Notice of Discharge

Are There Times When a HINN Is Not Appropriate?

HINNs must not be issued to patients who are:

Unable to comprehend the HINN

Under duress, in a medical emergency

In any case where the Emergency Medical Treatment and Labor Act (EMTALA) applies

What Is the Purpose of a HINN?

- Patients must be informed that they will be financially liable for services, except those services eligible for payment under Part B.
- Medicare beneficiary or representative must be issued a written form outlining the noncoverage including reason, appeal process, and cost of item/service.
- If proper HINN is not obtained, the patient cannot be held financially liable.

What Are the Conditions Included in the HINN Process?

- Regulation 42, CFR §412.42 (d) are: Item or service at issue must be diagnostic or a therapeutic service, medically unnecessary, and beneficiary must require continued hospital Inpatient care
- Inpatient stay must be covered
- Item/service must not be bundled into, or integral to, payment or treatment for diagnosis reasons related to the Inpatient stay

What Is the Value of the HINN Process?

Compliance with CMS	Increased patient satisfaction
Mitigate recoupment penalties	Mitigate denials
Improve bed management	Improve resource utilization

10.10 CMS Inpatient Only List (Addendum E) Tip Sheet

Inpatient-only procedures are those that CMS has determined providers must perform on an inpatient basis because they are invasive and require at least 24 h of postoperative recovery time or monitoring.

Providers should monitor the OPPS final rule in case CMS decides to remove more procedures. Addendum E is located in the CY2016 OPPS Addenda file listed under Related Links. This list is considered the Gold Standard used by most insurance companies in determining appropriate status for surgical procedures.

It is important to review the current CMS Inpatient Only list for Medicare beneficiaries having any procedure in order to ensure correct status and billing compliance

What Is the Difference with Other Resource Inpatient Only Lists?

Other resources have integrated inpatient surgical lists; however, they are often developed from billing and denial data. These lists are NOT the CMS Addendum E and may reflect only a single payor. The CMS Inpatient Only list is updated annually. Other resources may not be updated as frequently.

What Should Utilization Management Do When Reviewing Surgical Cases?

Validate payor source and for any payors that are not traditional Medicare FFS, verify the alignment with the CMS Inpatient Only list. Many commercial payors do not follow this list. Validate if any payor has a resource that should be referenced to determine procedures which they deem as inpatient.

Why Is the Inpatient Only List important?

Compliance with CMS	Mitigate denials
Improve reimbursement	Improve patient satisfaction

10.11 Transforming Episode Accountability Modes (TEAM) Tip Sheet

TEAMS aims to support better and more efficient care for beneficiaries. Cost-sharing for healthcare providers for 30 days of care post-discharge after the scheduled procedure

TEAMS is a Medicare program with the goal to reduce total episode costs and variation through the coordinated care of hospitals, physicians, and post-acute providers. The program rewards quality provided to traditional Medicare beneficiaries.

Is Participation in the TEAMS Model Mandatory?

CMS will implement TEAM in certain selected geographic areas to evaluate the effects of an episode-based payment approach on patient outcomes and Medicare expenditures.

CMS used a stratified random sampling method to select approximately 25% of eligible Core-Based Statistical Areas (CBSAs) to participate in TEAM. Facilities can also voluntarily participate.

What Patients Will Be Included as Part of the TEAM Model?

TEAMS includes five specific surgical episodes: Coronary Artery Bypass Graft (CABG), Lower Extremity Joint Replacement (LEJR), Surgical Hip/Femur Fracture Treatment (SHFFT), Spinal Fusion, and Major Bowel Procedures.

What Services Are Included in the 90-Day TEAM Model?

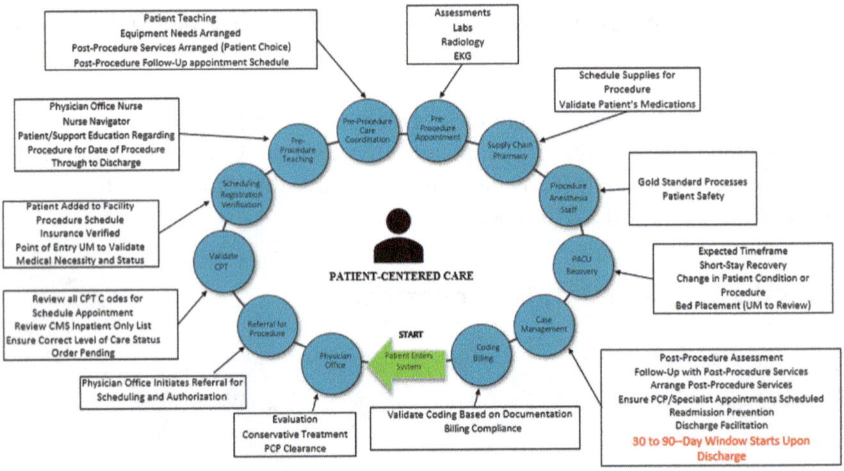

The interconnection of the different care providers and services involved in the care of the patients. Created by the author

What Is the Physician Role in the TEAM Model?

Physician engagement in the model is key to the success of the program. Many physicians are currently performing risk assessments during the evaluation of patients. Some physician offices are also initiating discharge planning with the patient and family prior to admission for the procedure.

What Is the Value of the TEAM Model?

Improve quality	Improve clinical care
Improve patient safety	Improve patient experience
Decrease cost	Improve resource utilization

10.12 Bundled Payments for Care Improvement (BPCI) Tip Sheet

The Bundled Payments for Care Improvement model aims to support better and more efficient care for beneficiaries admitted with one of 48 common DRGs. Cost sharing for all healthcare providers for 90 days of care.

> BPCI is a Medicare program with the goal to reduce total episode costs and variations through the coordinated care of hospitals, physicians and post-acute providers. The program rewards quality provided to Medicare Fee for Service beneficiaries.

What Patients Will Be Part of BPCI?

Patients identified to be included in the BPCI program are those with one of 48 DRG. Included are DRGs covering: Cardiac, Pulmonary, Renal, GI, Orthopedic, Neurology and Infectious Processes. For a comprehensive list visit: https://innovation.cms.gov/initiatives/bundled-payments/

What Services are Included in the 90-Day BPCI Program?

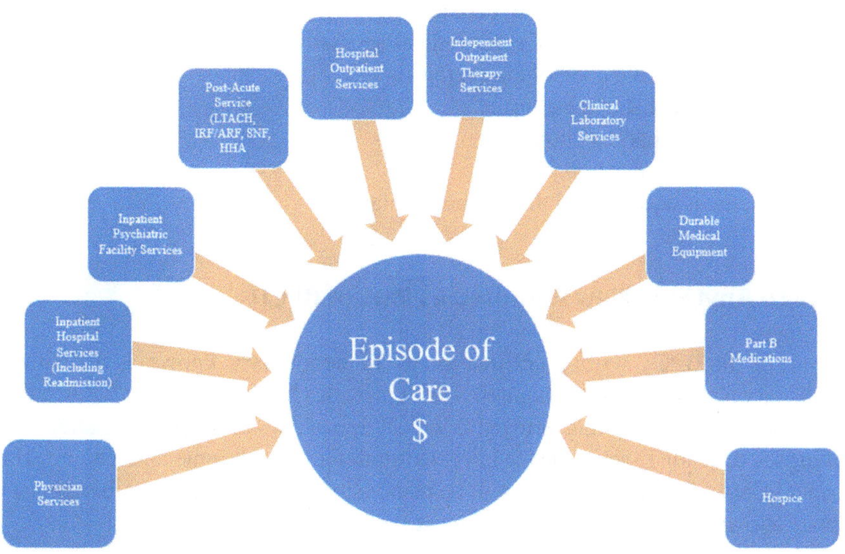
Post-Acute Service (LTACH, IRF/ARF, SNF, HHA
Hospital Outpatient Services
Independent Outpatient Therapy Services
Clinical Laboratory Services
Inpatient Psychiatric Facility Services
Durable Medical Equipment
Inpatient Hospital Services (Including Readmission)
Part B Medications
Physician Services
Hospice
Episode of Care $

The services included in the 90-day program. Created by the author

What Is the Physician Role in BCPI?

Physician engagement in the BPCI is a key to the success of the program. Many physicians are currently performing a risk assessment during the evaluation of patients. Some physician offices are also initiating discharge planning with the patient and family prior to admission for the procedure. Obtaining this screening information from the office will assist Case Management in addressing needs and concerns during the discharge planning process.

What Is Case Managements Role in BPCI?

Case Management plays an integral role in the BPCI program when comes to effective discharge planning.

Essential to the Success of the BPCI Program Is a Safe, Timely Discharge Plan

- Identify MD groups performing risk assessment
- Utilize physician risk assessment during planning
- Proactive discharge planning done within 24 h of admission
- Identify barriers to discharge
- Coordinate discharge plan with patient, MD, post-acute provider
- Ensure patient meets level of care medical necessity
- Consistently making and booking referrals
- Establish a safe discharge plan
- Obtain a signed patient choice letter
- Assist in obtaining medications
- Ensure care is coordinated throughout 90-day period

Is There Anything New Required as Part of BPCI?

As part of the BPCI, written notification to the beneficiary, known as the patient Beneficiary Notice or PBN, is required. This is provided by Patient Access/Registration during pre-admission testing or registration, at time of admission or immediately following the decision to schedule the lower extremity joint replacement procedure. The hospital Case Management team will be responsible for explaining the Beneficiary Notice and answer any questions regarding the BPCI.

What Is the Value of the Bundled Payment for Care Improvement Program?

Improve quality	Improve clinical care
Improve patient safety	Improve patient experience
Decrease cost	Improve resource utilization
Decrease readmissions	

10.13 Utilization Review Tip Sheet

Use of standardized criteria to evaluate patient medical records to demonstrate appropriateness of level of care and resources utilized for patients using evidence-based, objective criteria and supports the care provided for patients. Utilization Review nurses help healthcare providers implement informed care strategies that proactively and efficiently move patients toward health by ensuring that patients get the right level of care and the right care activities for the right amount of time.

Medical necessity is **defined** as accepted health care services and supplies provided to evaluate and treat a disease, condition, illness or injury and consistent with the applicable standard of care.

How Do We Use Information from a Utilization Review?

- Demonstrate medical necessity
- Proactive management of progression of care
- Manage length of stay
- Communication with payor

What Is the Review Process?

- Review all documentation available including: EMS, ED, provider, nursing, therapy
- Apply applicable and appropriate screening criteria
- Discuss with provider if additional clarification or documentation needed
- Engage Physician Advisor if needed for clinical determination
- Provide required medical necessity supporting documentation to the payor
- Follow for authorization or denial mitigation effort

What Is the Value of the Utilization Review Process?

Documentation validation	Improved revenue
Improve clinical care	Improve patient safety
Compliance with CMS Conditions of Participation	

10.14 Procedural Utilization Management Tip Sheet

Proactive management and appropriate intervention are essential to ensure procedural case are screened for correct level of care status pre-procedure and post-procedure to identify pertinent information supporting any potential changes in status to mitigate denials and positively impact revenue. This also supports length of stay and throughput which are crucial functions taking collaboration between Utilization Management and Care Management teams.

> Time is a critical factor in determination of status. Using the Medicare Two-Midnight Rule as a guide, patient's requiring less than 24–48 h of medical care are best managed at Observation level of care.

What Is Procedural Utilization Management?

The process of reviewing documentation to align medical necessity for procedures are performed at the right level of care based on the individual patient's medical needs and conditions and the payor authorization is aligned appropriately.

Screening medical documentation pre-procedure can identify patients who could potentially benefit from additional hospital level of care to optimize outcomes as an Inpatient. Early screening also leads to identification of patients appropriate for post-procedure interventions during the recovery period to allow them to return home at the end of their recovery period.

This takes collaboration and coordination between Utilization Management, physicians and their offices, patient access, insurance verification, therapy, and nursing to smoothly manage patients through the hospital.

What Can We Do to Manage Procedural Cases Optimally?

Review of documentation for individual patient needs	Utilize criteria to screen
Coordination with Physician Advisor	CMS 2MN Rule and medical necessity
Coordination with Revenue Cycle teams	Proactively communicate with payors

> **Utilization Management teams evaluate and optimize the utilization of healthcare resources and patient benefits while maintaining high-quality standards. Level of care is not one-size fits all.**

What Is the Value of Procedural Utilization Management?

Improved compliance	Decrease denials
Improve revenue	Improve patient throughput
Decrease delays in care	Improve patient experience
Improve bed management	Improve resource utilization

10.15 Concurrent Review Tip Sheet

Utilization Management performs concurrent review to proactively evaluate continuing hospital level of care needs and services for patients using InterQual and MCG criteria in partnership with the Physician Advisor. This information is shared with payors to **obtain appropriate authorization** in a timely manner to mitigate denials and impact the organization's financial stability.

> The role of Utilization Management is to provide standard, accurate, and current documentation of medical necessity to the payor to mitigate denials. UM is a liaison between the payor and the revenue cycle

What Is Concurrent Review Utilization Management?

An active process of reviewing documentation of patient care and progression in hospital treatment to validate appropriate level of care and communicate with the care team when patient is no longer meeting hospital level of care. This utilizes the patient benefits and hospital resources appropriately. The New England Journal of Medicine published research that demonstrated that patients hospital stays beyond medical necessity correlated with a 1% increase risk of a hospital acquired infection.

The role of regular concurrent review is to identify when a patient is progressed medically and ready to transition to the next level of care.

Concurrent review also takes a proactive role in reviewing documentation to provide to the payor to obtain authorization, or concurrently mitigate denials, to allow for timely billing.

What Can We Do to Manage Concurrent Cases?

Review of the medical record at a minimum of every 3 days

Coordination with Physician Advisor utilize criteria to screen

Communicate with CM for MDR Proactive management to facilitate care

Concurrent denial mitigation efforts are 66% more likely to be successful than retrospective appeal attempts

What Is the Value of Concurrent Review Utilization Management?

Mitigate denials concurrently	Proactive patient progression management
Improve revenue	Improve communication
Identify delays in care	Improve bed capacity
Improve resource utilization	Increase compliance with CoPs

10.16 Extended Stay Review Tip Sheet

Extended stay is defined as any case with a length of stay that exceeds 20 days over GLOS.

Managing the length of stay benefits the patient and the facility.

How Do We Manage Extended Stay Cases?

- Long Stay Rounds one to three times per week to discuss patient clinical progression, documentation and coding optimization, identifying transition of care needs and potential barriers.
- Meet with patient/representative frequently to discuss plan for stay and plan for transition of care, ensure patient choice is met for any post-acute provider services required.
- Utilization Management will continue to review cases for medical necessity using appropriate screening criteria every 3–7 days, or as required by payor throughout the stay.
- Extended stay cases will be presented to the Utilization Review Committee.
- At no time may a non-physician member of UR Committee make a medical necessity decision.

Why Do We Want to Manage Length of Stay?

Decrease payor denial rates	Decrease risk of hospital acquired conditions
Improve patient outcomes	Improve patient satisfaction
Improve patient throughput	

10.17 Emergency Department Utilization Management Tip Sheet

When Utilization Management in close communication and consultation with the ED, can provide guidance to ED providers on additional criteria to be met, further documentation and diagnostics needed on a case-by-case basis.

> Utilization Management offers knowledge the ED should be leveraging in understanding payor criteria and knowing how to appropriately classify patient status, whether for inpatient admission, observation, or discharge

What Can We Do to Improve ED Admissions?

- Active engagement with ED Providers
- Coordination with Physician Advisor
- CMS 2MN Rule and medical necessity
- Review documentation
- Utilize criteria to screen

What Can Utilization Management to for the Facility as Part of the Emergency Department?

Focusing on the front-end helps protect your bottom line, but it takes a real partnership between your ED and UR teams.

What Is the Value of Utilization Management in the Emergency Department?

Improved compliance	Decrease denials
Improve revenue	Improve patient throughput
Decrease delays in care	Decrease length of stay (LOS)
Improve patient experience	

10.18 Transfer Center and Direct Admit Tip Sheet

Approximately 1.5 million patients are transferred between acute care hospitals and approximately 15% of all non-elective hospitalization in the US come via direct admit. Proactive Utilization Management engagement at the point of entry will support reimbursement, patient status determination and facilitation of care.

The role of Utilization Management plays a pivotal role in ensuring patients receive appropriate care while managing costs effectively. It involves a systematic process of reviewing medical necessity, patient care, and service usage

What Is Role of Review Utilization Management?

Utilization Management performs initial review to proactively evaluate hospital level of care needs and services for patients using InterQual and MCG criteria in partnership with the Physician Advisor. These reviews assist accepting physician to determine appropriate level of care status and Utilization Management to initiate authorization communication with payors.

What Can Utilization Management Do to Support Transfer Center and Direct Admit Cases?

Review of the medical record reviewing for payor specific requirements related to placement

Coordination with Physician Advisor
Utilize criteria to screen
Building relationships with accepting providers
Communicate with CM for MDR and repatriation needs

Utilization Management ensures the best use of health care resources for optimal patient outcomes, proactive screening fosters quality care

What Is the Value of Utilization Management in Logistics Center and Direct Admits?

Proactive payor authorization initiation	Mitigate denials
Improve revenue	Improved communication
Improve bed capacity management	Improve resource utilization
Increase compliance with CoPs	

10.19 Observation Management Tip Sheet

Proactive management and appropriate intervention are essential to ensure Observation case are screened for correct level of care status and followed during progression of care to capture pertinent information supporting any potential changes in status.

This also supports length of stay and throughput which are crucial functions taking collaboration between Utilization Management and Care Management teams.

> Time is a critical factor in determination of status. Using the Medicare Two-Midnight Rule as a guide, patient's requiring less than 24–48 h of medical care are best managed at Observation level of care.

What Is Observation?

Observation status is provided to patients to ensure the care needed to manage your presenting illness or injury is appropriate which requires additional time, testing, diagnostics, or treatment to fully address the patient's needs.

Observation patients need to be identified early, particularly those with length of stay (LOS) approaching 2 days using EMR worklists or work queues. Collaboration and coordination between Utilization Management, Care Management, Nursing, Physicians, and other members of the Multidisciplinary Care Team is needed to smoothly progress the care of the Observation patients, which include appropriate conversion to Inpatient if needed to complete hospital care.

What Can We Do to Manage Observation Cases?

Review of medical record every 8 h to timely identify conversion or discharge readiness

Utilize standard screening criteria	Apply CMS 2MN rule correctly
Coordinate with Physician Advisor	Proactive discharge planning
Discuss progression in care during MDR	Identify delays in care
Facilitate completion of ordered care	Document barriers to progression of care plan

What Is the Value of Observation Management?

Improved compliance	Decrease denials
Improve revenue	Improve patient throughput
Decrease delays in care	Decrease length of stay (LOS)
Improve patient experience	

10.20 Outpatient in a Bed Management Tip Sheet

Proactive management and appropriate intervention are essential to ensure Outpatient in a Bed (OIB) case are screened for correct level of care status and followed during progression of care to capture pertinent information supporting any potential changes in status. This also supports length of stay and throughput which are crucial functions taking collaboration between Utilization Management and Care Management teams.

Outpatient in a Bed applies to patients who do not have acute medical needs necessitating hospital care, but, at the same time, are occupying a hospital inpatient unit bed.

What Is Outpatient in a Bed?

The goal is to clearly **identify these patients without medical necessity as soon as possible** and to **manage the patient until the appropriate transition** can be arranged.

- **Medical:** Patients placed in a hospital bed for medical conditions that do not have medical necessity for hospital level of care services
- **Social Admit:** Patient is placed in a hospital bed for the convenience of patient/family/doctor, often through the emergency department, while waiting for arrangements for an appropriate transition.
- **Procedural:** Patient is receiving outpatient treatments like surgery, cardiac cath lab, blood transfusion, hemodialysis, and/or chemotherapy and no other medical necessity is apparent.

Management of these cases is a fluid, ongoing process. Actively work to identify barriers to progression of care and develop strategies to overcome those barriers

What Can We Do to Manage Outpatient in a Bed cases?

- Review of the medical record upon bed request
- Utilize criteria to screen for potential Observation or Inpatient conversion
- Coordination with Physician Advisor
- Communicate with Case Management for discharge planning needs for OIB patients without medical necessity supporting admission and Multidisciplinary Rounds (MDR) discussion

What Is the Value of Outpatient in a Bed Management?

Improved potential revenue	Decrease unnecessary costs to patient
Improve communication	Improve resource utilization
Improve patient throughput Improve patient experience	

10.21 Physician Advisor (PA) Tip Sheet

Physician Advisors work in teams and are supported by the Utilization Management, Clinical Documentation Integrity, Case Management, and administrative team members. Each member of the Physician Advisor team works with the hospital in creating a strong relationship development.

> Physician Advisors should be well-respected by their colleagues, knowledgeable about admission criteria, medical documentation, and reimbursement, accessible, approachable, articulate and collaborative.

What Is the Physician Advisor Role?

- A physician review may be classified as: retrospective, concurrent, prospective, or peer to peer
- Medical necessity reviews that do not meet Utilization Management screening criteria
- Lack of progression of care
- Clarification or improvement education for physician documentation
- Denial from a payor for reimbursement support for Peer-to-Peer discussions or written appeal

What Does a Physician Advisor Do?

The Physician Advisors assist in providing a second level review of hospital cases to establish appropriate level of care determination, assist in denial mitigation and aid in patient progression through the hospital stay. The Physician Advisors provide a second physician review of the case and a peer-to-peer discussion, if necessary, with attending physician or payor physician.

A key component of the PA review process involves the Physician Advisors speaking directly with attending physicians. This collaboration helps the Physician Advisors gain greater understanding of the physician's intent, and also provides a peer-to-peer educational opportunity.

Physician Advisors provide a peer-to-peer discussion with payor physicians regarding concurrent and retrospective denials received.

What Is the Value of a Physician Advisor Program?

Improve quality of documentation	Decrease denials from payors
Improve communication	Improve patient care
Support hospital throughput	

10.22 Denial Management Tip Sheet

Authorization and certification issues drive a large portion of denials for care and treatment in the hospital setting. Improving documentation, providing clear communication, and developing a process to improve coordination between departments is needed to reverse the denial trends and obtain accurate authorization.

Denial of a claim is the refusal of an insurance company or carrier to honor a request for payment made by a hospital for health care services provided to a patient

How Can Utilization Management Prevent a Denial?

- Coordinate with Physician Advisor and Clinical Documentation (CDI) for documentation alignment Document concise medical necessity review including compelling quality statement to payor in a timely manner
- Communicate with payor to determine need for additional clinical information and to obtain continued authorization
- Document authorization information completely within the medical Communication throughout the revenue cycle teams

What Is a Concurrent Denial and What Can Utilization Management Do to Mitigate?

A Concurrent denial is a denial received prior to patient's discharge. It is important to document any attempts to overturn a denial appropriately. Utilization Management concurrent appeals activities are our first attempt to overturn the denial. **Research indicates that the best opportunity to mitigate a denial is while the patient is still in the hospital with a 66% increase chance of overturn**.

What Will Following a Denial Management Process Accomplish?

Standardize processes	Eliminate barriers
Reduce denial rates	Positively impact EBIDTA
Identify opportunities for process improvement	

10.23 Short-Stay Inpatient Management Tip Sheet

To ensure compliant and appropriate billing, Utilization Management is responsible for reviewing all Inpatient short-stay admissions to validate correctness for Inpatient billing. Escalation to the Physician Advisor may on occasion be necessary.

Reviewing short-stay Inpatient admission is important to ensure correct use of patient benefits and compliance with billing practice. UM clinical knowledge is necessary to validate the Inpatient status.

Is the Inpatient Level of Care Billing Valid?

CMS Inpatient Only Procedure (for payors following this list)	Left Against Medical Advise (AMA)
Initiation of mechanical ventilation	Expiration
Transfer to another acute care facility	Transition to comfort care, palliative care or hospice services
Inclusion of prior midnight(s) spent receiving care in an outpatient setting including the ED or outpatient procedural area (add Occurrence Span Code 72 to account)	

What Is the CMS Policy Regarding Length of Stays Expected to be Less than Two Midnights?

- For stays for which the physician expects the patient to need less than two midnights of hospital care (and the procedure is not on the Inpatient Only list or otherwise listed as a national exception), an Inpatient admission may be payable under Medicare Part A on a case-by-case basis based on the judgment of the admitting physician. The documentation in the medical record must support that an Inpatient admission is necessary, and is subject to medical review.
- CMS is reiterating the expectation that it would be unlikely for a beneficiary to require Inpatient hospital admission for a minor surgical procedure or other treatment in the hospital that is expected to keep him or her in the hospital for a period of time that is only for a few hours and does not span at least overnight. CMS will monitor the number of these types of admissions and plans to prioritize these types of cases for medical review.
- No change for stays over the tow-midnight benchmark.

What Is the Value of Reviewing Short-Stay Inpatient Accounts?

Mitigating denials	Validating appropriate billing status
Compliant billing practices	Patient satisfaction
Proper us of patient benefits	

10.24 Interrater Reliability Tip Sheet

Standardized audits performed to evaluate compliance of policy and procedure and regulatory requirements as a patient moves through the continuum of care.

Interrater reliability: In statistics, interrater reliability, interrater agreement, or concordance is the degree of agreement among raters.

What Is Reviewed Using Interrater Reliability?

Level of care	Concurrent review
Medical necessity documentation and criteria	CMS 2MN Rule and medical necessity
Initial review	Quality of documentation
Use of Physician Advisor	Application of criteria
Discharge assessment	Discharge planning/Care coordination

Why Is the Interrater Reliability Audit Performed?

Ensure accuracy
- Demonstrate quality of documentation
- Confirm completion of required work
- Validate timeliness of documentation

What Is the Value of Interrater Reliability Audits?

Meet CoP in treating all patients with the same care

Standardize approach to work	Process improvement
Documentation improvement	Improve quality of care
Mitigate denials	

10.25 Care Coordination Tip Sheet

The purpose of Care Coordination is to proactively identify and resolve barriers that impede the progression of care and decrease length of stay. **CMS Regulations** require Care Coordination as part of the Condition of Participation to be compliant with the Affordable Care Act, Bundled Payments, CJR and the Readmission initiative. (CMS - ACO Quality Measures #8-13).

What Is Care Coordination?

Care Coordination involves the **assembling of personnel and other resources needed** to carry out all required patient care activities and is often **managed by the exchange of information among participants** responsible for different aspects of care. The goal is to ensure the ***right*** patient receives the ***right*** treatment at the ***right*** time for the ***right*** reason in the ***right*** location with the ***right*** outcome at the ***right*** cost.

The role of Care Coordination is to ensure the deliberate organization of patient care activities between two or more participants (including the patient) involved in a patient's care to facility the appropriate delivery of healthcare services

How Can We Coordinate Care for Our Patients?

- Focus on **evidence-based, patient-centered outcomes**
- Identify **high risk patients** early
- Facilitate **communication** across the continuum of care
- Help ensure **comprehensive care planning**
- Ensure **appropriate sequencing and continuity** for the patient's plan of care
- Act as **an advocate** for the patient
- Manage **patient length of stay** appropriately to reduce avoidable/denied days

Who Is Part of Care Coordination?

The Interdisciplinary Team: Patient, Physician, Pharmacy, Nursing, Respiratory Therapy, Case Management, Physical/Occupational/Speech Therapy, and Dietary. Working together ***WE*** can improve the quality of care for our patients and the outcomes they experience.

What Is the Value of Care Coordination?

Increase patient satisfaction	Improve patient safety
Improve the patient experience	Improve quality of care
Increase communication	Decrease delays
Decrease denials	Reduce health care costs
Improve patient transition between levels of care	

10.26 Multidisciplinary Rounds (MDR)/Patient Progression Rounds (PPR)/Interdisciplinary Team (IDT) Tip Sheet

The **multidisciplinary health care team** includes a diverse group of members (e.g., physicians, psychologists, social workers, and occupational and physical therapists), depending on the needs of the patient.

What Is the Purpose of the MDR?

To promote quality patient care, promote efficient use of available health service resources, to coordinate care to improve outcomes, patient throughput and positively impact quality of medical care and to increase communication and coordination between hospital departments.

> Multidisciplinary team is a group of health care professionals from diverse fields who work in a coordinated fashion toward a common goal for the patient.

Who Are the Participants in the Multidisciplinary Team?

Attending Physician	Nursing	Administration
CaseManagement	Laboratory	Therapy (PT/OT/ST)
CDI	Patient Access	Pharmacy
Financial Counselors	Radiology	Dietary

What Does the Multidisciplinary Team discuss?

Patient progression of care	Patient needs	Discharge needs
Patient authorization	Avoidable delays	

What Is the Value of the Interdisciplinary Team?

Coordination and teamwork	Improved quality of patient care
Improved patient throughput	Improved satisfaction

10.27 Resource Management Tip Sheet

Resource Management is a formalized program that focuses on the utilization and consumption of healthcare resources.

What Is Resource Management?

Management of healthcare related costs to ensure resources utilization is matched to the patient's acuity and severity of illness, eliminate inefficiencies in the delivery of care and optimize cost efficiency and quality of care.

An emphasizes an ongoing, systematic process that assists the healthcare team in improving performance and patient care outcomes that decreases health care costs.

What Areas Are included in Resource Management?

Pharmacy
Diagnostic Testing
Equipment
Level of Care Assignment
Patient Throughput
ICU Rounding
Respiratory Therapy
Supplies
Nursing Activity
Time of Discharge
Use of Protocols

What Is the Value of Resource Management?

Improve quality of care
Optimize length of stay
Eliminate inefficiencies
Improve patient throughput
Process improvement
Mitigate denials

10.28 Discharge Planning Tip Sheet

"The hospital must have in effect, a discharge planning process that applies to all patients" per CMS (§432.43). The Discharge Planning screening includes functional status, living arrangements, risk assessment, and support contact information. All of these areas are necessary to meet the Conditions of Participation requirement.

A well-executed discharge plan assists the patient by creating a smooth and safe transition and aids the patient in achieving their individual goals of care after discharge.

- The discharge planning information provides an overall picture regarding the patient's current needs and the needs at the time of discharge.
- Communicate with the Interdisciplinary team regarding needs and plan of care to ensure safe discharge for patients.
- Evaluate the patient's existing resources and care needs.
- Evaluate new needs based on the patient's current medical condition.
- Document the risks to a safe discharge, placement needs and expected discharge date for the patient to ensure development of a plan which alleviates the risks and creates a smooth and safe transition for the patient.

What Is the Value of Discharge Planning?

Increase effective planning	Increase patient satisfaction
Increase communication	Decrease readmission rates
Increase patient safety	

10.29 Discharge Planning: Home Health (HH) Tip Sheet

Home health care is a wide range of health care services that can be provided in your home for an illness or injury. Home health care is usually less expensive and more convenient than the care you receive in a hospital setting.

> Home Health care is clinical medical care provided by a registered nurse, occupational therapist, physical therapist, or other skilled medical professional and is often prescribed as part of care following hospitalization.

What Can Be Managed by Home Health Care?

- Wound care for pressure sores or a surgical wound
- Patient and caregiver education
- Intravenous or nutrition therapy
- Injections
- Monitoring serious illness and unstable health status
- Physical, occupational, respiratory and speech therapy
- Ambulate safely in the home with appropriate assistive device with supervision/minimal assistance of caregiver
- Able to transfer safely with supervision/minimal assistance of caregiver
- Patient is homebound due to functional or medical status

What Should Be Expected from Home Health Care?

- Doctor's orders are needed to start care. Once your doctor refers you to home health services, the home health agency will schedule an appointment and come to your home to talk to you about your needs and ask you some questions about your health.
- The home health agency staff will also talk to your doctor about your care and keep your doctor updated about your progress.
- It's important that home health staff see you as often as the doctor ordered.
- Check what you're eating and drinking.
- Check your blood pressure, temperature, heart rate, and breathing.
- Check that you're taking your prescription and other drugs and any treatments correctly.

- Assess your progress and current health condition.
- Check your safety in the home.
- Teach you about your care so you can take care of yourself.
- Coordinate your care. This means they must communicate regularly with you, your doctor, and anyone else who gives you care.

What Is the Benefit of Home Health?

Regain independence	Encourage self-sufficiency
Slow decline in overall health	Partner with hospital
Reduce readmissions	

10.30 Discharge Planning: Hospice Tip Sheet

Hospice care tries to provide the best quality of life for dying patients. This is done through a holistic approach. It offers spiritual, mental, emotional, and physical comfort to the patients, their families, and their caregivers. The main goal of **hospice** care is to reduce potentially unavoidable physical, emotional, psychosocial, and spiritual suffering encountered by patients during the dying process.... Rendering support to the patient, their families, and caregivers with the overwhelming physical and psychological stresses of a terminal illness.

> People often wait too long before seeking hospice care. Often in the US hospice is not provided until the last week of life losing the opportunity for quality of life.
> A hospice team is a group of people who understand the specific goals of hospice care.

What Qualifies for Hospice Care?

Determined to have a terminal illness (which is defined as having a prognosis of 6 months or less if the disease or illness runs its normal course;

Not have made a hospice election, and

Not previously received the pre-election hospice services

What Services Are Offered by Hospice?

- Comfort care for pain and symptom management
- Maintenance care for existing chronic conditions such as diabetes or emphysema
- Support for emotional, social, psychological and spiritual needs and issues related to dying

- Needed drugs, medical supplies and equipment
- Mentoring for the individual, his or her family, and friends on best practices in patient care
- Services like speech and physical therapy, which can be accessed when needed
- If receiving hospice at home, payment for short-term inpatient care is available when symptoms become too much to manage or when caregivers need a respite break to take care of themselves
- Grief counseling is available and can take the form of a support group, one-to-one therapeutic counseling, spiritual counseling, phone check-in calls and educational materials for surviving family and friends.

Where Can Hospice Services Be Provided?

At patient, family, or friend's home	In a free-standing hospice center
In a hospital	In a skilled nursing or assisted living center

What Are the Benefits of Understanding Hospice?

Familiar environment	Comprehensive care plan
Provide a sense of dignity	Decrease financial burden
Provide family support	Personalized care and support

The Improving Medicare Post-Acute Care Transformation (IMPACT) Act of 2014 modified the Social Security Act requiring that SNFs be required to submit data for public reporting. In response, the Centers for Medicare & Medicaid Services (CMS) established the SNF QRP and authorized the Secretary to report quality measures that relate to care provided by SNFs on a CMS website (*Find Healthcare Providers: Compare Care Near You | Medicare*)

The benefit of a Skilled Nursing Facility (SNF) is the access to skilled medical professionals 24/7. This healthcare team can provide services that are critical to residents' well-being.

What Patients Benefit from Skilled Nursing Facility Level of Care?

- Skilled nursing care included short-term rehab services, such as medication management, therapy and nursing interventions, to help patients recovery after illness, injury or surgery
- To quality for skilled nursing care, the patient must needs services that cannot be provided at a lower level of care, and they must show potential for improvement
- Medicare Part A covers skilled nursing care for up to 100 days in each benefit period, but only for short-term rehab after a qualifying hospital stay (3 days)

What Are the Key Purposes of Skilled Nursing Facilities?

- SNF serve as a step between a hospital stay and returning to the prior living setting, offering therapies such as respiratory, physical, occupational, and speech therapy to help patients regain strength and function
- 24-h medical professional care delivery including IV medications, injections, complex wound care, and management of chronic, exacerbated, or terminal conditions
- Activities of daily living (ADL) assistance

What Is the Difference Between SNF and Nursing Home Placement?

SNF are short-term facilities with a goal of helping the patient regain their ability to do activities of daily living such as bathing, dressing, cooking, personal hygiene, walking, and getting into/out of a bed or chair. be available to them

A nursing home is a long-term residential center primarily for patients who are medically stable but can't be cared for at home due to chronic conditions or a lack of mobility. Residents at a nursing home may not need 24/7 intensive care, but medical assistance is available if the need arises.

What Are the Benefits of Understanding Skilled Nursing Facilities?

Improve functional independence	Improve quality of life
Improve cognitive & communication skills readmission	Reduce hospital readmission

10.31 Discharge Planning: Acute Inpatient Rehabilitation (IRF/ARF) Tip Sheet

Acute Inpatient Rehabilitation Hospitals offer an intensive therapy program focused on helping patients recover from serious illnesses, injuries, or surgeries. It involves a team of medical professionals, including physicians, nurses, and therapists, who work together to help patients regain their ability to perform daily tasks and achieve functional goals.

Acute Rehabilitation hospitals focus on helping patient regain independence in performing daily tasks and achieving functional goals. The healthcare team provides education and support for recovery.

Regain independence	**Encourage self-sufficiency**
Slow decline in overall health	**Partner with hospital**
Reduce readmissions	

What Patients Benefit from Acute Inpatient Rehab Level of Care?

- Patients recovering from stroke, brain injury, spinal cord injury, amputation, and other serious conditions.
- Individuals who need intensive therapy to improve their ability to perform daily activities like dressing, bathing, and walking.
- Patients who require specialized medical care and supervision during their recovery.

What Are the Requirements for Acute Rehabilitation Services?

- Intensive Therapy including physical, occupational, and speech therapy services, patient ability to tolerate 3–4 h of therapy daily
- Physician oversight by a physician specializing in physical medicine and rehabilitation (physiatrist)
- 24/7 nursing care
- Care coordination

What Diagnoses Meet CMS Criteria?

• Stroke	• Amputation
• Brain Injury	• Active osteoarthritis in 3 or more weight-bearing joints
• Spinal Cord Injury	• Rheumatoid arthritis: active and involving multiple joints
• Neurological disorders such as MS or Guillain-Barre Syndrome	• Systemic vasculitis with joint inflammation after failed OP treatment
• Femur Fracture	• Major trauma
• Lower Extremity joint replace (only if bilateral, BMI >50%, or >85 years old	• Congenital deformities

What Are the Benefits of Understanding Acute Rehab?

Improve functional independence	Improve quality of life
Improve cognitive and communication skills	Reduce hospital readmission

Long-Term Acute Care Hospitals play a very important role in health **care**. Our hospital accommodates patients that often have very few alternative options. They are critically ill and/or have multi-system complications or failure which require hospitalization for an extended period of time.

10.32 Discharge Planning: Long Term Acute Care (LTAC) Tip Sheet

LTAC(H) focus on patients with severe illnesses and multiple medical conditions that require ongoing, intensive care beyond the capability of Skilled Nursing Facilities helping lift the burden of long-stay complex patients from the acute care hospitals.

What Is Managed by Long-Term Acute Care Level of Care?

- Vent Weaning / Respiratory Therapy 24/7
- Cardiac Monitoring
- Long-Term Antibiotic Therapy
- Wound Care (vacs, grafts, flaps, complex wounds)
- Biomedical Debridement
- Nutritional Support (TPN)
- Dialysis
- Medication Titration (Drips)
- Ancillary services (lab, radiology, etc.)
- Education for patient and family
- All levels of hospital care: Medical, Surgical, Telemetry, Intermediate and Intensive Care

Regain independence **Encourage self-sufficiency**
Slow decline in overall health **Partner with hospital**
Reduce readmissions

What Are the Requirements for Long-Term Acute Care Services?

- Requires medical practitioner assessment and/or intervention daily
- Treatments cannot be provided at a lower level of care
- Requires skilled services 6 or more hours per day
- Ventilator dependent 6 or more hours per day, including weaning
- Requires minimum 30 days of medical treatment

What Are the Benefits of Understanding LTAC?

Improve resources utilization Improve readmission rates
Improve patient throughput Decrease revenue loss
Extend continuum of care for complex patients

10.33 Length of Stay Alphabet Tip Sheet

As with all areas of healthcare, Length of Stay has its own scrabble pieces which can be arranged differently. Understanding each acronym is the important first step to optimizing the length of stay for our patients.

> The goal of Length of Stay Optimization is to meet the clinical needs of the patient without placing them at increased risk.

What Is Length of Stay Optimization?

Discharge too early and the patient is at risk of readmission. Discharge too late and the patient is at risk for contracting a hospital acquired condition. We are challenged with finding the balance to optimize the healthy outcome for our patients.

What Are the Acronyms and What Do They Mean?

L O S	**Length of Stay:** The period of time a patient remains in a hospital
A L O S / T L O S	**Acute/Actual/True/Raw Length of Stay:** The current period of time a patient has been in the hospital.
G M L O S / G L O S	**Geometric Mean Length of Stay:** A statistical/mathematical term that is applied to determine the expected length of stay for a patient population with the same diagnosis.
D R G	**Diagnostic Related Group:** Used to classify patients for the purpose of reimbursement.
C M I	**Case Mix Index:** A relative value assigned to a DRG used to determine allocation of resources to care for and treat the patients in that group.
C C / M C C	**Complication or Comorbidity/Major Complication or Comorbidity:** Secondary diagnosis which prolong the length of stay and/or affect treatment.
D I Graphic created by author	**Discharge Index:** Total number of hospital discharges divided by the total census.

10.34 Length of Stay Tip Sheet

Improving and reducing length of stay (LOS) improves financial, operational, and clinical outcomes by decreasing the costs for the patient and improve outcomes by minimizing the risk of hospital-acquired conditions.

> A long average length of stay can often indicate poor coordination of healthcare services and delayed decision-making, resulting in unnecessary hospital waits and early discharges.

Why Does the Hospital Want to Optimize Each Patient's Length of Stay?

- Each day in the hospital confers an ~1% risk of hospital acquired infection www.nejm.org/doi/full/10.1056/NEJMoal306801#t=articleResults
- Results of a study at the VA found reducing LOS by 1 day decreases mortality by 25% and ~3% readmission reduction www.adviory.com/daily-briefing/2012/12/19/researcher-shortening-hosital-stays-may-improve-outcomes
- Discharging patients at the national average (GLOS) is an opportunity to increase the financial success of the facility
- Improves patient throughput for all patients across the continuum of care
- Improved ED throughput

How Can We Optimize Length of Stay?

Long-stay/Complex Case Rounds

Team: Physician lead, Case Management, therapy, CDI, and nursing
Focused review: Cases >GMLOS, length of stay >6 days
Discussion: Clinical readiness for transition to level of care status, hospital
Identify: Barriers to discharge and optimized coding for clear expected length of stay goal

Who Is Needed for a Partnership to Assist with Throughput?

Post-Acute providers from all levels are necessary to facilitate patient throughput and impact length of stay. Either formal or informal partnerships with Home Health, Skilled Nursing Facilities, Acute Rehabilitation Facilities, and Long-Term Care Hospitals are important.

KEY: regardless of partnerships, patient choice MUST drive discharge provider selection.

Regain independence	Encourage self-sufficiency
Slow decline in overall health	Partner with hospital

10.35 Length of Stay Optimization Tip Sheet

The principle motivation for reducing LOS was to improve quality and outcomes for patients. Ensuring that patients are the focus of efforts led to different and better decisions than if the focus is primarily on financial or operational outcomes.

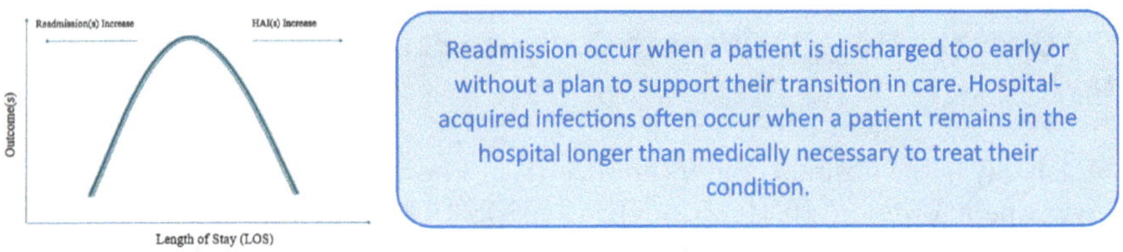

This image shows the optimal length of stay to prevent readmission and also minimize development of a hospital acquired condition. Created by the author

How Can We Optimize Length of Stay for Each Patient?

Define discharge planning process: anticipate discharge and communicate planned discharge date and plan
Track each patient's clinical progression: ensure entire team is on the same page
Executive support and engagement: necessary organization or process changes
Prioritize labs and diagnostics: communicate with ancillary departments for early testing/procedure
Reduce delays in admission from ED: ensure each patient receives appropriate care as soon as possible
Assess current discharge practices: work effectively with team schedules and available resources
Reduce patient wait time between care activities: most inpatients spend too much time waiting for care
Schedule procedures on an outpatient basis if appropriate: provide services in the most appropriate setting
Engaged and educated physician staff: as part of the care team, physicians are included in planning and scheduling
Know discharge barriers: post-acute service availability, transportation, processing orders

What Is a Process for Reviewing Extended (Outlier) Cases?

Long-stay/Complex Case Rounds

Team: Physician lead, Case Management, therapy, CDI, and nursing
Focused review: Cases >GMLOS, length of stay >6 days
Discussion: Clinical readiness for transition to level of care status, hospital
Identify: Barriers to discharge and optimized coding for clear expected length of stay goal

What Is the Benefit of Length of Stay Management?

Decrease risk of HAI	Decrease readmission rate
Raise employee satisfaction	Increase patient satisfaction
Boost patient engagement	Improve facility processes

10.37 Avoidable Delay/Day Tip Sheet

Timely, accurate documentation of Avoidable Days and Delays assist in identification of opportunities to positively impact length of stay, readmission rates, and guide development of process improvements to address the root causes of these days/delays.

> Identification of root cause(s) of delays in patient care or additional avoidable days leads to positive impact on patient care and development of improved processes.

Why Do We Document Avoidable Days/Delays?

Identify specific factors contributing to avoidable days. This allows for tracking of specific causes of a denial or delay and any interventions done by Case Management, to develop a proactive plan to address the issues and reduce the denials and delays in patient care.

Identify Medicare cases for review of self-denial/Part B billing.

Where Is Information Regarding Avoidable/Denied Days Documented?

Document the process and any actions taken by Case Management to facilitate throughput of patients including facilitation of testing, treatments, evaluations, and discharge to avoid a delay in progression of the patient's care. Documentation should include the root cause details within the facility EMR or other identified location.

What Documentation Should Be Included?

Root cause reason	Root cause attribution

Who Receives Documentation?

Report during Utilization Review Committee meetings for management

Provide to the Medical Staff Office for use in FPPE/OPPE reporting for individual providers

Identification of process improvement opportunities	Improve communication
Identification of scheduling/staffing needs	Improve efficiency and quality
Establish new leading practice standards	Identify potential patient risk
Compliance with Conditions of Participation	

10.37 Readmission Management Tip Sheet

Section 3025 of the Affordable Care Act added section 1886(q) to the Social Security Act establishing the Hospital Readmissions Reduction Program, which requires CMS to reduce payments to IPPS hospitals with excess readmissions, effective for discharges beginning on October 1, 2012. The regulations that implement this provision are in subpart I of 42 CFR part 412 (§412.150 through §412.154).

For patients, hospitalizations can be stressful; even more so when they result in subsequent readmissions. While many readmissions are unavoidable, researchers have found wide variation in hospitals' readmission rates, suggesting that patients admitted to certain hospitals are more likely to experience readmissions compared to other hospitals.

What Is a Hospital Readmission?

A hospital readmission occurs when a patient is admitted to a hospital within a specified time period after being discharged from an earlier (initial) hospitalization. For most payors, this time period is defined as 30 days, and Medicare includes hospital readmissions to any hospital, not just the hospital at which the patient was originally hospitalized. Medicare uses an "all-cause" definition of readmission, meaning that hospital stays within 30 days of a discharge from an initial hospitalization are considered readmissions, regardless of the reason for the readmission.

What Are the Impacts of Hospital Readmissions?

- Financial
- Quality Rating
  - Example: Readmissions account for 22% of the quality star rating for the facility

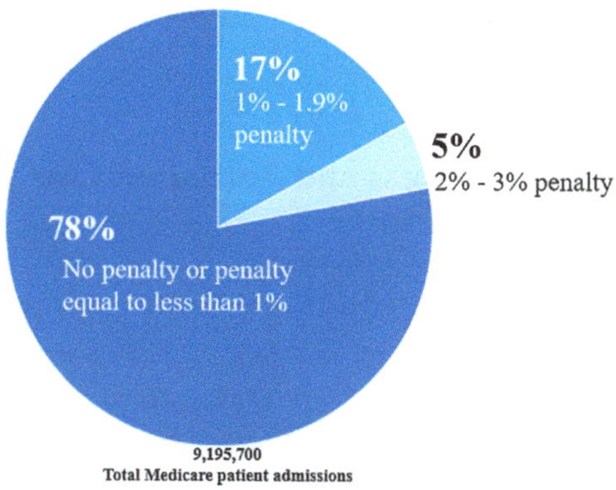

Graphic created by author

How Can Readmission Rates Be Lowered?

- Clarifying patient discharge instructions
- Assess each readmission for root-cause and improve process to prevent the cause
- Ensure patient is provided with appropriate resources
- Coordinating with post-acute care providers and patients' primary care physicians
- Reducing medical complications during patients' initial hospital stays

What Is the Value of Reducing Readmissions?

Increase revenue	Improve quality
Decrease penalties	Improve communication
Development of Accountable Care Organizations	

10.38 Supporting Patients with Behavioral Health Issues Tip Sheet

Hospitals are associated with experiences of illness and suffering, although they *have* been known to resolve people's problems and even help to produce rather good outcomes like successful births. However, the overall perception for most people is that of large edifices, highly technological and elaborate, not readily comprehensible and rather overpowering. Becoming a patient is therefore usually associated with stress, consisting of Lazarus' (1966) three components: *threat*, fear of the unknown; *loss*, freedom and familiar surroundings; and *challenge as* to how one is going to cope with hospitalization

Stress caused by a visit or admission to the hospital and the care associated with treatment in the hospital may hinder patient recovery and, in some cases, it may cause potential life-threatening psychological changes.

What Causes Increased Stress and Decreased Coping in Patients with Behavioral Health History?

- Long waits
- Increased noise
- Perceived lack of personal safety
- Sensory overload
- Limited access to necessities
- Unfamiliar sounds, sights and smells
- Sleeping in a strange bed/room
- Changes in normal routine
- Confrontation

How Can We Reduce Stress for This Population?

Identify and reduce stressors
Provide basic and accurate information
Intervene when patient is distressed
Move to quiet area, speak softly
Provide reassurance
Discuss expectation for treatment
Decrease noise, if possible
Group treatments together if possible

Regain independence
Slow decline in overall health
Encourage self-sufficiency
Partner with hospital
Reduce readmissions

11 Conclusion

Learning Objectives

1. **Commitment to Continuous Professional Development:** Recognize the importance of ongoing education and training for Case Managers to stay current with best practices and evolving healthcare standards.
2. **Empower Patients Through Advocacy:** Identify ways in which Case Managers can empower patients by providing information and resources, enabling informed decision-making and promoting patient-centered care.
3. **Contribute to a Thriving Healthcare System:** Discuss how effective Case Management can improve overall patient outcomes and contribute to a dynamic and resilient healthcare system.
4. **Embrace a Vision for the Future:** Reflect on the collective effort required in Case Management to drive positive changes in the healthcare system, emphasizing compassion and innovation.

As we pause to reflect on the profound and transformative role of Case Management within the healthcare system, we are reminded of the critical importance of this vocation. Case Managers serve as the essential link between patients and the complex web of healthcare services, embodying the core values of advocacy, compliance, and ethical patient care. Their unwavering commitment to upholding patients' rights ensures that individuals receive not only competent and appropriate care but also the dignity and autonomy they rightfully deserve throughout their healthcare journey.

As we advance into this promising future, the role of Case Managers will expand in response to evolving healthcare technologies and methodologies. Their ability to adapt and integrate new practices will be crucial in maintaining the equilibrium between innovation and patient care. With the advent of telehealth and digital platforms, Case Managers are now equipped with powerful tools to monitor and support patients

S. Garceau, *Interdisciplinary Case Management: A Nursing Practice Approach*,
https://doi.org/10.1007/978-3-032-20960-3_11

remotely. This technological evolution does not replace the human touch but rather enhances it, ensuring that care is continuous and accessible.

The emphasis on preventive care and early intervention is another area where Case Managers can make significant strides. By identifying potential health issues before they escalate, they can implement strategies that minimize hospital admissions and improve overall patient wellness. This proactive approach not only benefits patients but also reduces the strain on healthcare systems, allowing resources to be allocated more efficiently.

The integration of interdisciplinary teams highlights the collaborative nature of modern healthcare. Case Managers work alongside doctors, nurses, social workers, and other professionals, fostering an environment where diverse expertise converges to address patient needs comprehensively. This teamwork underscores the importance of communication and shared goals in delivering holistic care.

Education and continuous professional development remain pillars of effective Case Management. As healthcare standards evolve, so too must the knowledge and skills of those who navigate its complexities. Continuing education programs, certifications, and training workshops ensure that Case Managers remain at the forefront of best practices, ready to tackle the challenges of tomorrow with confidence and competence.

The significance of mental health in the overall well-being of patients cannot be overstated. Case Managers, often acting as patient advocates, are in a unique position to recognize and address mental health concerns, coordinating with mental health professionals to provide comprehensive care. This integrated approach acknowledges the interconnectedness of physical and mental health, promoting recovery and resilience.

In the realm of patient advocacy, Case Managers empower patients by providing them with the information and resources necessary to make informed decisions. This empowerment fosters a sense of autonomy and respect, aligning with the fundamental principles of patient-centered care. By advocating for patients' rights and preferences, Case Managers help create a healthcare environment where patients are seen, heard, and valued.

As we continue to pursue excellence in healthcare, let us recognize the indispensable role of Case Managers in shaping a future that blends compassion with cutting-edge innovation. Their dedication to patient care, compliance, and continuous improvement is the bedrock upon which a thriving healthcare system is built. Together, we can forge a path towards a future where every patient receives the highest standard of care, and every Case Manager is equipped to lead with empathy, expertise, and unwavering commitment.

The journey ahead is one of collective effort and shared vision. By embracing the transformative power of effective Case Management, we can elevate the standard of care, improve patient outcomes, and foster a healthcare system that is as dynamic and resilient as the people it serves. It is through our combined efforts that we will ignite a movement for positive change, shaping a brighter future for all.

FSC
www.fsc.org
MIX
Papier | Fördert gute Waldnutzung
FSC® C083411

Kolibri 360 GmbH
Ferdinand-Jühlke-Straße 7
99095 Erfurt, Deutschland
produktsicherheit@kolibri360.de